Your Life Isn't Over - It May Have Just Begun!

A Mini-Manual for Managing Diabetes

REBECCA HENSLEY

committed2change
unlimited

Cover and author's photographs: Crystal Boatenreiter
Book layout and cover design: Pattie Steib

ISBN: 1515068056
ISBN-13: 978-1515068051

Printed in the United States of America

10 9 8 7 6 5 4 3 2 1
First Edition

I am not a medical professional of any kind and do not claim to be one. I am only offering information that I have gleaned from my own experience with managing diabetes over the past seven years.

The contents of this book are not intended as a substitute for professional medical advice, diagnosis, or treatment. Always seek the advice of your physician or other qualified health provider with any questions you may have regarding diabetes or any other medical condition. Do not disregard professional medical advice or delay in seeking it because of something you read in this book.

For Joy –
who told me I would figure it out
(thank goodness, you were *right*!)

and

to the thousands who will be
diagnosed diabetic today:
may this book make
your road easier

Acknowledgements

If I were to try to say thank you to everyone who played a role in the ultimate production of this piece of work, the resultant addition would be longer than the book itself. The list would have to include everyone who knew I was a writer before I did (all the way back to my third grade teacher, Mrs. Vogt). It would have to include everyone who looked out for me when I was making less than rational decisions or I wouldn't have lived to write anything (the ones who lived to tell the tale know who they are and might not want to be mentioned). It would have to include those who helped me get through grad school (or I might never have believed I could take on and finish any project this ambitious). And it would have to include all those who contributed financially to the set up process. They more or less forced my hand. Once they contributed, I had to finish it. (Thank you, thank you, thank you.)

I thank Crystal Boatenreiter for the photographs that captured my vision of myself so beautifully. I thank Pattie Steib for jumping in with both feet and treating me with respect as if I wasn't a rank beginner, which helped me to rise to the occasion. And above all, I give my undying gratitude to my friend and colleague Dayne Sherman, who has been shamelessly pushing me to publish for years, told me how to do it, taught me how to do it, and then walked me through the process as if he was personally invested (while also doing the same for so many others). Everyone should have such a friend.

Preface

Let's face it. Being told you definitely have diabetes – of any type – is a head butt. Nobody wants to hear they have a terminal illness. Let alone that no one knows exactly how specific individuals get it or exactly what will work for specific individuals to manage it so it doesn't kill them.

I get it.

As a matter of fact, I've *got* it.

But over the past seven years, I've actually gotten *more* fit, *more* energetic, *more* positive in my way of looking at things, and even *cuter* (though I've obviously gotten older – and I wasn't that young to begin with).

Not everything that works for me will necessarily work for you. Some things I don't include in this book because they *haven't* worked for me *would* work for you. But you have to start somewhere. And this book isn't for children, so somebody with a different set of experiences is going to have to cover that waterfront.

I may be very different from you in various ways. And the particular type of diabetes I have (which some doctors call Type 1.5) is not precisely like other types. You may never have to take insulin, for example, while I had to start taking shots last summer after six years of managing my disease with diet, exercise, and oral medications.

So what's the point of writing this at all? It's that there's hope.

Whatever you're feeling right now, whatever your challenges are, I can guarantee you that I've had to face enough of them at one point or another that I've learned some tips that could very likely benefit you – especially if you're new to this party. This means that, if you read this little book, you won't have to figure out every single thing for yourself.

I'm not going to pretend that this book has all the answers you'll ever need. But I can promise you that, if you'll read it with an open mind, by the time you finish it, you'll feel less like jumping off a bridge than you did when you opened the cover.

Along the way on this journey I never imagined I'd be taking, I've had some tough days emotionally from time to time. Some depression. Some anxiety. Some frustration. And some discouragement. But think about it now – wouldn't I have had all those same emotions with or *without* diabetes? I had lived long enough before I was diagnosed to know that a life without diabetes is not a charmed life by any means.

On the other hand, a life **with** diabetes is, as you may already know, complicated, even when it's good. And there's a ton of information out there – at doctor's offices; in hospital diabetic education programs; in videos, magazines, and books; and all *over* the internet, where you will find (if you haven't already) *so* much information (and some of it contradictory) that your brain could implode if you try to make sense of it all at once.

Some of it is so scientific as to be virtually useless to most of us. Some of it is so simple, it amounts to common sense. And some of it won't have anything to do with your type of diabetes or your life circumstances – or at least not yet.

That's where this book comes in. It's not real long. It's not written in scientific jargon. In fact, I hope it reads like a conversation between two diabetics sitting across from each other in comfortable chairs on a patio somewhere, sipping iced coffee on a beautiful summer day.

So, if you've just been diagnosed with diabetes or you're just coming to grips with it after spending some time refusing to accept it and get on with the process of being happy *anyway*, you may find some helpful hints in here. One thing's for sure: your life isn't over. It *may* have just begun. Isn't it worth taking the time to find out?

Introduction

I remember it like it was yesterday. I went in for my annual physical check-up in February of 2008, not expecting anything out of the ordinary, feeling perfectly fine (or thinking I did). I had just moved to the area six months before to take a position teaching at a university in a small town in Louisiana. I didn't know my new doctor, but he seemed personable enough and was a good looking, youngish family practitioner, so I was completely unprepared for his clipped and somewhat dark announcement.

Walking into the exam room with my file in his hands, he said, "Your glucose is a little high. I want you to go to a lab for a glucose tolerance test."

It didn't really grab me much at the time. At sixty-two years of age, I had had my share of dealings with other doctors, had undergone a few surgeries, including an early hysterectomy and having my gall bladder removed a couple of years before. But, typical of physicians, who seem to like to hold the news until they have all the facts, he didn't explain why he wanted me tested further and certainly did not prepare me for the test.

When I arrived at the lab on the morning in question, hungry from fasting all night until the appointment, a young woman who clearly did not have adequate training for the task had me drink eight ounces of a liquid that was supposedly fruit-flavored, but fairly awful tasting. And then, every hour for three hours, she drew my blood.

The way I feel about needles, I would have hated the process, in any case, because my veins (I have been told by medical professionals) are small and likely to roll. And roll they did that morning. The woman stuck me over and over and over in three different harrowing episodes. She showed only minor frustration as she dug the needles around in the flesh of my already bruising forearm, and I was coming to understand that, if this was the test, then I should *probably* be concerned about why it had been ordered.

Sure enough, when I returned to my doctor's office for the results, he breezed into the room and announced simply, "I was right. The glucose tolerance test came back positive. You have diabetes."

I don't think I would have been much more surprised if he had told me I had bubonic plague. Diabetes doesn't run in my family. Wearing a size fourteen, I wasn't particularly overweight. I had been drinking soy milk, eating whole grain bread, and taking vitamin supplements for decades. I always took the stairs instead of the elevator. I didn't feel sick (though the fact is that I was having diabetic symptoms and didn't even realize it: a dry mouth, occasional blurred vision, and multiple trips to the bathroom in the middle of the night to drink water and pee).

Still, while I was admittedly on the back side of sixty, I had more energy than anybody else I knew over forty. How could I possibly have what he called a "terminal disease?" Surely, the diagnosis was incorrect. A doctor had done an angioplasty on me shortly before, discovering to his chagrin that the inside of my heart was perfectly healthy. Couldn't this be the same way, my brain was screaming, while my ears heard the doctor say casually, "Managing this condition will be like having a second job."

My brain took a second step backward. *Really?* I was already working twelve-hour days as a full-time instructor. How could I handle *more* responsibility? And what did he mean by that anyway? I left his office reeling with a handful of paperwork and instructions to see a diabetic educator and a diabetic nutritionist. For starters.

Part of my horror had to do with the fact that I had moved to Louisiana only six months before to fill a nine-month temporary position. Did this diagnosis mean

I was dying? Would I be bed-ridden soon? Would the university decide not to move me into a more permanent position, if they learned of my new situation? And what in the world would I do without health insurance if they let me go? How the hell did this happen to *me*?

The diabetic educator was a pretty blond named Debbie who maintained eye contact with me across the little desk like she was talking someone down off a ledge on the twenty-second floor.

"You didn't do anything *wrong*," she kept repeating in a reassuring voice. "We don't *know* what causes it. And especially in cases like yours..."

I panicked even worse than I had at the doctor's office and quickly spiraled into an increasingly dark and even desperate abyss. Having been raised in fundamentalist Christian churches, though I had stopped attending as a young woman, the belief system is never far from the surface. Was I being punished for some reason? If so, this was too harsh. I hadn't done anything worthy of a *death* sentence. How could I possibly have wound up with a "terminal disease" when I had never felt stronger or more capable? I felt as if I was finally, really coming into my own personally and professionally. And now *this*!

I was shortly moved to another room where I met Virginia, the nutritionist, a highly trained and matter of fact speaking woman who described a complex system of foods I could and could not have and a monumentally complicated process of when and how much to eat, with dire consequences if I didn't follow the rules religiously. I listened, took notes, went home, and somehow got through the semester.

I didn't tell anyone because I was convinced that if the department found out, I would not be made permanent. I couldn't miss a lick at work or someone might start asking questions. And I couldn't face my deepest fears about my newly discovered condition when I had to use every ounce of my strength just to meet the daily requirements of living.

One day when I had a question about some disease-related matter, I called Debbie to talk. This was one of the services offered at the local hospital system and I was using it on a regular basis. On this particular day, however, she wasn't in her office and I wound up speaking with someone else – equally trained and competent, I'm sure – but unknown to me and, in my fragile emotional state, I couldn't deal with the change.

"I don't know exactly what would work best for you," the unknown diabetic educator – whose name was actually Joy – said, "but *you'll* figure it out."

I fell apart. I raved. I wept. I even attacked her over the phone.

"*How* am I supposed to figure it out?" I ranted. "I was only told I *have* this disease two months ago. You've all told me it can *kill* me if I don't do the right things. And now you're telling me you don't know what the right thing *is*, but that *I'll* figure it out! What if the diabetes kills me before I can *do* that?"

When the semester finally came to an end, I lay down on the floor in a fetal position in the tiny apartment I had rented while I was waiting to find out if I was going to have to find another job in yet another town. Weeping freely now, I presented myself to the Universe in abject surrender.

"I can't *do* this," I wailed. "And I don't know how to *handle* it!"

Then I remembered the principles and coping mechanisms I had learned during two decades of recovery from drug addiction. I already *knew* how to manage a terminal illness – one day at a time!

I got up off the floor, wiped my eyes, and hit the internet to learn more about my new self. Now, seven years later, I have indeed learned that managing my diabetes has become for me very much like a second job. It can be frustrating. And it can be frightening. But most of the time now, it's just one thing about myself that I choose not to ignore. It is what it is.

Just as Joy predicted, over the past seven years, I have indeed figured out a lot of stuff about living with diabetes. Stuff that makes my life easier. Stuff that has helped me get and stay healthier than I would have been if I hadn't developed diabetes. And even stuff that allows me to feel "normal" and enjoy the life I've been given.

I go through changes once in a while because of some aspect of my disease, and life – of course – is life. But in general, I'm comfortable and happy, even with this monster following me around like a ten thousand pound pet elephant. If you want to know how I'm doing it, keep reading.

Part 1

Mindblown

Looking back now, I'm not sure I exhaled once during the first six months after my diagnosis. My focus on what I believed I must do and not do was absolute. Virginia, the nutritionist, had asked me a lot of questions about how and what I normally ate, declared that I would have less trouble than some because I had a lot of fairly decent eating habits already, and then crafted a regimen just for me. I was to eat 45 grams of carbohydrate first thing in the morning and then another 30 grams of carb every few hours for the rest of the day: mid-morning, at lunch, mid-afternoon, and at dinner time, with a few carbs just before bed[i]. I followed it like I thought my head would fall off if I failed to do so.

In the effort to simplify the process, I quickly found routines I could work with. Breakfast wasn't much of a problem once I got used to knowing what my portions had to look like. The mid-morning and mid-afternoon snacks consisted generally of nuts and fruit or a low carb chewy granola bar. I didn't have time to think about anything more complicated when I was running from class to class on my job as a teacher. Dinners were usually lean meat and salad or veggies. But lunches caused me some duress. No more lunches in the student union. No more Popeye's chicken or deep dish pizza slices. And I soon relegated myself to a daily Lean Cuisine selection.

This was not as slam dunk a solution as it may sound. While the brand touts itself as "Lean," the "Cuisine" was not always lean *enough* for my carb allotment. Reading the carbohydrate grams listed on the back of the various boxes, I soon learned that some of the selections had as few as 20 grams of carb (yay!), but some (the same size and not appearing necessarily to be vastly different in the picture on the box) had as many as 54 grams of carb, nearly *twice* what I was allowed. The result, needless to say, was that I had to learn exactly which selections I could have and stay away from the rest. It didn't take long before this became tiresome and self-pity began to rear its ugly head.

On one trip to the grocery store, as I wheeled my cart down the frozen food aisle to the Lean Cuisine section, I reached for the door handle and burst into tears. I suddenly had visions of myself eating the same little lunches every day for the rest of my life and I just couldn't face it. It wasn't *fair*, I wanted to tell somebody, as if that would change anything.

"You better get a *grip*!" I growled at myself, opening the door. "You're not *suffering*! In a world where 34,000 children will die today for want of food or water, you'll eat *six times*."

It was my first realization on my new journey and an important one.

* * * * *

Just because I can't have everything I want doesn't mean my life isn't worth living.

* * * * *

There are millions of folks in the world – even just down the street, if I could see behind closed doors – who would probably love to trade my "problem" for one of their own. That doesn't make my problem easy to live with, but there's no point in whining if it's not going to solve anything. And in the great scheme of things, diabetes is *not* the worst thing that ever happened to a human being on the face of the earth.

So I grabbed my lunches, reminding myself that I was lucky to have a job, lucky to have the money to purchase the lunches, lucky to be able to figure out what was best for me, lucky to be motivated to do what would help me stay alive, and lucky to know I was lucky! I haven't cried in the grocery store since.

As the days turned into weeks and the weeks into months, though, other issues became as trying as eating the same things over and over. For one thing, I got the idea somewhere that I couldn't have coffee anymore (and most certainly not those sugary, topped-with-whipped-cream-and-sprinkles-delights they sell at Starbuck's). Fancy coffee was how I kept my hellified schedule on track. Now, not only was I operating on "slow" all the time, but the social ritual of "going for coffee" with students and colleagues was now closed to me. I thought.

Even after I learned that I could give up the herbal tea for coffee again, when I liked, I still missed the loss of what I *really* wanted at Starbuck's and other such stores. Until, that is, I overheard someone at a coffee counter in a bookstore order a cappuccino with sugar-free mocha syrup and half and half[ii].

"What did you just order?" I queried, so excited I wasn't even embarrassed to be asking a rank stranger a personal question.

When the customer repeated himself, I did a quick mental tally and turned to the young person behind the counter. "I'll have one of those, too," I said enthusiastically.

As I sipped my creamy, chocolaty, hot coffee drink with a level of satisfaction probably wildly disproportionate to its importance, I learned another truth that has stood me in good stead since that time.

* * * * *

Just because I can't have what "everybody else" has doesn't mean I can't have delicious.

* * * * *

I learned to call it "doing my homework" when I asked to see the Starbuck's nutrition information, a little folder most restaurants keep for people to look at or even take with them. Shortly after this experience, I learned that many restaurants and even fast food joints also have that information on the internet. So I looked up the places represented on the campus and found something I could order at each of them without blowing my game plan. There might only be one option, but it was on there. What that meant was that if I was with other people or craving Taco Bell, I wouldn't want to order a five-layer burrito like I used to (at 65 grams of carb), but I *could* have a Gordita Supreme with chicken (at 29 grams) accompanied by a diet soda and not feel left out.

Seven years later, this all seems a little frantic, but at the time, these baby steps kept me saner than I would have been, if I had continued to go around believing that all joy was gone from my life forever. Admittedly, one gordita and a soda is not a lot of food, but it's a pleasant change from a Lean Cuisine, especially if eaten at a sociable table with friends.

As I got used to eating less (and I *did* get used to eating less without feeling that I was going to starve), I began to notice something I had never paid attention to before. Other people (it seemed now) were eating a *lot* more food than they probably needed. Keep in mind that I live in Louisiana – a state that prides itself in the enjoyment of food and drink as a cultural lifestyle. But as I began to change my habits along those lines, I began to notice how some – maybe even many – of the folks around me were wildly unhealthy: severely overweight, drinking alcohol to excess, and often smoking cigarettes on top of it all.

Their skin was pasty. Their clothes bound their bodies as if they were about to split their seams. They wheezed as they walked to their cars in the parking lot. They ate much more than me, but seemed to enjoy it less. And I began to realize that they just ate like that because they were used to doing it. For all the brouhaha about enjoyment of life, they didn't appear to be happy with the way they felt or the condition of their bodies.

"I need to (give up cigarettes, go to the gym, lose ten pounds...fill in the blank)," they would say as they stuffed down their super-sized fries on top of the bacon double cheeseburger and enough soda to float a small dinghy, not meaning it and knowing I wouldn't expect them to.

I didn't say anything, of course. It was none of my business. I couldn't even suggest that they might wind up diabetic – like me – since Debbie has made such a point of saying that we don't *know* why people develop the disease. But something unexpected was taking place in my head now that I was eating better. My body felt different and that feeling changed even more when I started hitting the gym.

They had told me that exercise would help me keep my glucose under control, but there was so much to process and getting on top of the food requirements (not to mention my emotions) was all I could handle initially. But when my birthday showed up about six weeks after my diagnosis, I gave myself a present of some sessions with a student fitness trainer. I don't think I was very serious. In fact, in retrospect, I think I was just doing it because they told me to. At my age, I didn't have any expectations that I would "get in shape" or anything. In fact, I was concerned that I might embarrass myself by passing out or injuring myself on a machine. I felt ridiculous in my workout clothes while the bulk of those at the gym could easily have been my grandkids. But, as it turned out, people in a gym are there for a reason and if you're there to work out, they give you props.

As I continued to show up, however, (largely because I had paid for it), I slowly but surely began to make progress. It's true I never compared to the twenty-year-old women athletes putting themselves through their paces to please a coach. But whereas I could only do a few exercises at first, in time, I could do more and then more. And by the time I returned to see the diabetic educator and the nutritionist six months after my diagnosis, I had lost forty-eight pounds and had the beginnings of what can only be called a not very impressive, but certainly evident "six-pack" of muscles in the middle of my abdomen.

Who knew that was even *possible*?

When I walked through the door for my appointment, Debbie looked startled. "You must be borderline *underweight*!" she exclaimed. "Stop losing!"

"I don't know if I *can*," I responded seriously, not getting the point of her concern and feeling that I had somehow done something wrong in spite of all my efforts.

"Why *not*?" she queried, alarmed. "What are you doing?"

"What you *told* me to," I promptly replied.

At which point, she stopped, mesmerized, tipped her head to one side, and said, "You *are...*?"

Turning toward another doorway, she called out to Virginia to come see, saying to her pointedly as she entered the room, "She says she's doing what we *told* her to do..."

Virginia was clearly as flabbergasted as

Debbie had been. And then they explained the reason.

"*Nobody* does what we tell them to," they said, shaking their heads sadly.

Apparently, as a rule, when people are diagnosed with diabetes, they typically see the diabetic educator and the nutritionist as their new worst enemies, two people who can eat whatever they want, but have been put into the patient's life for the express purpose of tormenting them, denying them their favorite foods and drinks, and robbing them of their joy.

These newly diagnosed diabetics never call for input on how to handle their new requirements. They resent and resist the practices they've been instructed to follow. They miss appointments. And when they make them, they *swear* they eat almost nothing and cannot *imagine* why they haven't lost a pound.

Here I was, down forty-eight pounds in six months and you would have thought I was a prize-winning poodle. They were grinning from ear to ear as if I had done it just to please them.

"May I give you a hug?" Virginia said wistfully. "Most patients hate us. It's nice to have one come in like you."

The thing is, it hadn't occurred to me before that minute, but I never blamed the messengers. If it wasn't *my* fault that I had developed diabetes, it certainly wasn't the *doctor's*. It wasn't the educator's or the nutritionist's fault either. It didn't make them *happy* to give me tough news or suggest that I would now need to do one thing or another. They were telling me what I needed to know to live long and well. Why would that be a *bad* thing?

Here I was, with a life-threatening disease, and instead of just being left to my own devices to do the best I could, my health insurance was providing a whole medical team to keep me alive: a doctor, an educator, a nutritionist, a lab I'd be visiting *often*, and the list would get longer and longer as time went on. I had more help than I knew what to do with!

When my primary doctor eventually called me "a poster child for diabetes," I realized he must be dealing with the same issues. "You're the only diabetic patient I have," he told me at one point, "that manages their condition the way you do. You'd be surprised at how they refuse to listen, *even* when they wind up in the hospital over and over."

But hiding from the truth doesn't change the truth. And getting mad at a medical professional for trying to save your life makes no more sense than sticking a knife in your inner tube when it's the only thing standing between you and drowning. And whether I like it or not,

* * * * *

Denial doesn't make it so.

* * * * *

As the years unfolded, I managed my attitude and my behaviors related to my condition increasingly well most of the time.

One of the principle reasons for this was that I kept reminding myself what would happen if I didn't.

When friends say, "Oh, my **gosh**! I would **never** be able to do what you do!"(as if I have a *reasonable* choice not to), my answer is immediate and uncompromising. "It's not so hard," I say casually. "I just weigh my options."

Then, holding my hands out in front of me, palms up, I look from one hand to the other to demonstrate the process: "Sweet tea." (I look to the left); "Being able to see." (I look to the right). Sometimes, just for good measure, I repeat it again, indicating each hand as I do.

"Sweet tea."

"Being able to see."

It's actually a no-brainer. But I'm not really trying to convince them. I'm reminding myself. It *is* a no-brainer. I *love* sweet tea, but I haven't had a single glass of it since I was diagnosed. Quite simply, there is no sweet tea in the world that tastes *soooo* good, I'd be willing to trade my sight for it. Blindness is just *one* of the complications that can occur when a person with diabetes doesn't control their glucose levels. And complications can occur whether I manage my disease or not. But I'm not going to make *sure* they happen.

---

[i] This was based on my height and weight and on what I was used to eating. Obviously, if you're six foot two, weigh 185, and work as a roofer, the diabetic nutritionist is going to recommend more carbs for you than I could have. So keep that in mind as you read this book.

[ii] When crafting your own delicious custom coffee beverage, forget about the whipped cream and sprinkles, but most coffee shops have a range of sugar-free syrups. Try them one at a time until you find your favorite. (Some people, for example, like a blend of sugar-free hazelnut and sugar-free vanilla which makes a tasty French Vanilla option.) Coffee shops that offer flavored coffee give you the option of asking for "Southern Pecan flavored coffee with sugar-free caramel syrup" or "English Toffee flavored coffee with sugar-free vanilla syrup," etc., if you like. Additionally, half and half actually has less grams of carbohydrate than whole milk which has less carbs than skim and you need a lot less half and half to lighten your coffee than either of the others – besides it tasting richly decadent. So you might want to keep that in mind. It's not like you're drinking it by the glassful. A cappuccino, by the way, has 12 grams of carb and a latte has 18, but regular coffee with sugar-free syrup and half and half only has about 4. And it took me years to learn all this. You're welcome.

Part 2

Weight, Weight – Don't Tell Me!

The fun part of losing all that weight was that I was suddenly as cute as a bug. I went from a size 14 to a size 4 and occasionally even a size 2. Now, that might not mean much to you guys, but ask a woman what a size 2 is and she's going to tell you, it's what fourteen-year-old girls wear if they're anorexic. I didn't wear a size 2 in middle school. In fact, before I wore a size 2, I wondered what kind of Barbie dolls actually wore those little tiny clothes. Certainly not grown women!

But here I was with the "problem" of trying to find jeans in a size 2 that didn't have rhinestone studs reading "Foxy" on the pocket or intentionally ripped out knees. Most of the slacks that fit me at that point were hip-huggers and, while I could wear them, I was more than a little past wanting to. Still, I was enjoying my new body.

Walking across the campus in my size 2 jeans, I felt downright smug. Thanks to the drop in weight and the workouts I was doing, I could go up the stairs in my building with less effort than my students. And when I would catch a glimpse of myself in one of the plate glass windows at the Student Union, I would strut my stuff like a runway model.

Friends and even students complimented me daily on how good I looked in those jeans, that long sweater, that cocktail dress, and I would respond, "Well, they diagnosed me as diabetic last year, so there's got to be *some* kind of up-side to having a terminal illness! I guess this is my reward for having no choice."

The fact was, I had unlimited choices.

All kinds of them. I could *not* watch what I ate. I could *not* go to the gym. I could *not* run around the house over and over before work in the morning with the big dog I had brought home from the shelter one day. But I didn't want to die. I didn't even want to start having complications. If being cute in my jeans was the payoff I got, that was nice and all, but I was enjoying being alive and I didn't intend to give it up before I was damn good and ready.

When my daughter complained one day that she was having a hard time dropping ten pounds that she wanted to get rid of, I offered a suggestion.

"Do what I did!" I told her, trying to be helpful. "I followed the regimen my health team gave me and the pounds just *melted* off with no effort at all."

"But, Mom..." she scoffed, "*you* were afraid for your *life*. Most of us don't have that kind of motivation."

It occurred to me that she was exactly right. And I was caused to think of a line I read in a pretty good book[i] I found on the internet. It made the point that if you want to live a long and healthy life, you should get a terminal illness because then you'll do all the stuff *everybody* ought to do, but doesn't. Of course, I was also coming to realize that most people with diabetes (which *is* a terminal illness, after all) don't do the stuff everybody ought to do either. In fact, many of them don't do the stuff they're told they must do to *survive*, which I found hard to understand.

As the months and years went by, I learned that there are so many diabetics in this country that my primary doctor, who's not even a specialist, has to stay on top of all the latest research on the topic because he has so many patients with the disease. And this was borne out in my daily life when I would casually mention my condition and *often* discover that the person I was speaking to – young or old – was also diabetic. Or their child was. Or their mother. Or their boyfriend. And almost no one (but me and selected celebrities and the people writing the magazine articles I was reading) was making any real attempt to "manage" their disease.

I was puzzled. I wasn't suffering. In fact, I was running around feeling cute. I had started discovering little treats I could work into my food plans. I had gotten over the shock of learning about my diagnosis. And my life had stabilized back into a more or less normal existence. So why did so few others want to make any attempt to do the same thing, I wondered.

I imagined them saying things like, "Well, everybody's got to die of *something*." Or "My grandfather smoked cigars all his life and lived to be one hundred with no sickness at all. So I just think we're all different." Or "I could be careful *every day of my life* and then get run over by a bus." Or "If I'm going to give up everything I love, I might as well be dead."

But I couldn't get past the complications issue. I know everybody's going to die (even me) and I could get run over by a bus on any given day. But I don't want to lose my sight or my feet or my ability to get around. In other words, my quality of life is about more than sweet tea. Or biscuits and gravy. Or ice cream sundaes. All of which I love.

My quality of life is about being happy enough to laugh and healthy enough to have sex[ii]. I enjoy being able to hold down a job so I can buy stuff I want and take care of my needs. I want to continue being useful and hanging out with friends and taking road trips and being surprised by life – in wonderful ways – for a good long time yet. And if I don't get cut down by a bus, I'm likely to, even *with* diabetes *if* I manage it.

Apparently, many folks with diabetes are so overwhelmed by the idea of "managing" their diabetes, they won't even try. But it doesn't have to be all that scary if you just keep a few things in mind.

First of all, throw out the rage with the garbage. (And those Moon pies you think you can't live without. You can. Way better than you can live without your feet.) I mean, who are you going to be mad at anyway? The doctor? Your body? Life? God? All those people who can still eat Moon pies?

When I first met her, I was pissed at my nutritionist. She was pudgy and pleasant and not diabetic. So while she was describing in great detail what the rest of my life should be like at dinnertime, I would be looking at her and thinking that *I* was thinner than *she* was and how come *she* could have whatever she wanted while I'm counting my peanuts – none of which had anything to do with what we were talking about.

There are a gazillion things I could be dealing with right now that would be horrible to face or imagine. But all I have is diabetes. And as un-fun as that is (as I said before) it is *not* the worst thing that ever happened to a human on the face of the earth. Further, being angry enough to self-destruct the rest of my good days over it makes no sense at all. For me to decide that if I can't have *everything* just the way I want it, I will throw away every good moment, every beautiful memory, every lovely relationship I ever had or ever *will* have would reduce me to the maturity level of a two-year-old being told to go to bed when she wants to play. Am I going to refuse to have **any** joy because I can't have **only** joy? Am I going to trade years and years of a rich and satisfying life for a few ice cream sundaes – that will be accompanied by trips to the hospital and living with terror and putting my family through anguish? What am I willing to lose to have sweet tea? Absolutely *nothing*.

I could make a list of all the terrible things I've had to live through in my life. You'd be impressed. They've been many and pretty awful. The point is: I lived through them. Just like you lived through the trials and tribulations with which **you've** already dealt. I tell my students that there *is* life after weird. And they laugh. But they get what I mean.

I could also make a list of all the good

stuff that came my way. It's funny how easy it is to forget the good stuff when something happens to me I don't like, though honestly, dealing with diabetes has actually helped me to develop a more level-headed approach to such things. I tend not to freak out as fast or as much as I used to. It makes my glucose level rise, for one thing, and that's not good. But I also like going through my own life acting like a grown-up, sailing through situations with some suave, knowing that others (especially younger people) have begun to see me as a person who's cool under fire. I'm not so sure I would ever have reached where I am now if I hadn't had the extra pressure of a terminal illness to give me some perspective. So I've come to see this as another perk of having this "problem."

With or without diabetes, however, I'm surrounded by beauty. There's a mason jar of zinnias on the corner of my desk. There's a photo of my daughter peeking around the edge of my laptop. There's a thank you card that reads, "You're the best" standing up next to my internet modem where I can see it. And a glass paperweight I picked up years ago on a trip to the Bahamas. And all *that* is right in front of me where I sit this minute. Not bad, huh?

When push comes to shove, though, I personally had far less rage than fear. When I first heard the diagnosis. Whenever my glucose was high. Or low. When I had reactions to changes in my medications. When I spent an entire summer worrying about growing old. And eventually, when I was trying to figure out how to get my brain around the necessity of taking insulin for the rest of my life. Fear, in fact, become my worst nightmare. Because fear could make my glucose rise, too, and make it harder to problem-solve[iii], and, if I wasn't careful, spiral into depression,

Six years after my diagnosis, when an endocrinologist put me on insulin and I crashed and burned all over again, when I was presented with a whole new set of diabetic challenges with no notice whatsoever, when I was trying to figure out how to go on with my life, if that was even possible, I read the story of Supreme Court Justice Sonia Sotomayor, who was born into a poverty-stricken Puerto Rican family in the Bronx and had to stand on a chair so she could boil her own syringes on a stove when she was seven. And right then, she became my diabetic Patron Saint. If she could do that and grow up to be a Supreme Court Justice, I could shake off my panic long enough to make peace with some medical technology she could only have dreamt of when *she* started out.

---

[i] The First Year: Type 2 Diabetes: An Essential Guide for the Newly Diagnosed by Gretchen Becker and Allison Goldfine (Da Capo Press, 2006) is written by a nurse who has been living with diabetes for decades. Every other chapter is made up of fairly understandable explanations of the scientific realities of diabetes, which is a good thing if you can handle it and are ready for that level of information. If you're not, you can just skip those chapters your first time through the book.

[ii] Don't pretend you're shocked. I plan on enjoying sex until I'm too old to remember what it is. And though I've read that diabetic men sometimes develop erectile dysfunction, that's not necessarily a symptom of diabetes, from what I understand, but rather can be a complication of not managing their disease. Which is certainly something to think about.

[iii] The term for figuring out why your diabetes and your body are interacting in a negative way.

Part 3

Diabetes Boot Camp

In an industrialized society, we're all familiar with the term "jump start." We jump start a car when it's acting sluggish. We jump start a career with some training, some tools, or a new set of clothes to help us get the job. And we jump start a tour in the military with a few months at boot camp. But being told you're diabetic comes as such an unwelcome and unexpected surprise, we tend to freeze up. Time stands still. Everybody else in the world seems to be bustling around us as if we're invisible. And no matter what we do, this diagnosis is going nowhere[i].

A lot of the information coming at us when we're first diagnosed just falls into an abyss of shock. We hear the words, but we don't compute the meaning. And any pressure from a medical professional or a loved one is likely to meet belligerent resistance. Like Dorothy whirling in a tornado and then being dropped unceremoniously in Oz, we have no idea where we've wound up and what will happen next. We just know we're not in Kansas anymore.

They do enough blood tests on us to bleed us dry. They give us stacks of sheets full of detailed instructions. And we try to understand so we can fit it all into the lives that we still must live one way or the other. But it's complicated.

I knew I needed to find out what my blood glucose was first thing in the morning, but I didn't want to stick my finger and bleed before my eyes were fully open. Still, I did it. And that was only one of what seemed like a thousand new rituals I needed to embrace on a daily basis. The thought that I was going to have to hurt myself like that millions of times before I died was daunting and, from what I can gather, lots of people don't do it.

After all, you don't necessarily feel bad until you're in real trouble. So if you don't stick your finger and test your blood to find out what your glucose numbers are, you can just pretend nothing is wrong. Right? For me, that equated to playing Russian roulette. I might get away with it for awhile, but there would eventually be a consequence for this behavior that I wanted even less than the finger pricks. So I made an important decision at that point that I've pretty much stuck by ever since: not to get into an argument I can't win.

The American Diabetes Association reports that, in 2012, 21 million people in the United States (nearly half of them over 65 years of age) were already diagnosed with diabetes and that an average of 4,657 *additional* people are diagnosed with this condition daily. It is either an underlying or contributing cause of death for 300,000 of us every year. And whether we like it or not, if we've already been diagnosed, we are faced with an argument we can't win. Either we will accept the situation and work to manage it or it will produce complications that will kill us: high blood pressure, heart attacks, strokes, and/or kidney disease, not to mention the amputations and blindness that may plague us for years first. A pretty grim scenario.

When I was finally told I would have to begin taking insulin, I turned a somber face to the endocrinologist and said in a serious voice something along the lines of: "Okay, doctor, can you make a prediction about how long I may have left?" I was thinking that, if I was now going to have to take insulin, I must surely be closer to dying than I had ever been before.

He made no attempt to hide his alarm at my question when he responded, "It's not the *diabetes* that kills you! It's the *complications*!"

"Ohhhh," I said, getting his point immediately. "You mean, the insulin can help me to control my glucose levels...and, as long as I manage my glucose levels,...I'm less likely to develop complications...so I'm more likely to be okay."

In other words, if more than 20 million of us have already been diagnosed diabetic and "only" 300,000 (less than 2%) die annually, that means that the other 98% of us can – just like Supreme Court Justice Sonia Sotomayor – live with this disease quite well, some of us for multiple decades. So I'm playing the odds. And how I do that is what this little book is about.

It may or may not be particularly helpful to you or your loved one, depending on how similarly situated we are. I had a fairly good health insurance plan when I was diagnosed, for example, so I was able to get my medications, supplies, and other treatment without going too deeply into my pocket[ii]. I had a full-time job, which meant that I could purchase the healthy foods I needed to be buying. Because I teach at a university, I could belong to the fitness center or even hire a personal trainer for an affordable fee. I already knew how to do research on the internet to access the masses of information available and chat rooms where other diabetics could be found holding discussions day and night. And I am a constant reader. I ordered and read books, read websites[iii], and unapologetically snatched up piles of magazines in doctors' offices and marched out with them as if I didn't realize they were still in my arms.

If your circumstances are different from mine, you may have to engineer some alternate solutions. Medicare, for example, is covering millions of diabetics over the age of 65, including free medication and testing supplies. Even the small town I live in has several programs for senior citizens that offer various types of fitness opportunities daily for free or nearly free and are advertised in the local newspaper. And besides books on diabetes, most public libraries provide computers connected to the internet and many offer free computer training for beginners. The magazines at the doctors' offices are also free, of course – if you beat me to them.

My point is that the odds are with us, if we manage our disease. And we can manage it without being rich, if we do the work. But a jump start is a good idea and can propel us into a good level of momentum. At least it did for me.

I didn't quibble with the Diabetes Monster. I walked out of the doctor's office on Day 1 of my new life, drove to the pharmacy to pick up my new medications and supplies, and entered Diabetes Boot Camp before nightfall. My boot camp lasted about six months and was centered around four areas: (1) testing my glucose levels by placing a drop of blood on a test strip stuck into a glucometer first thing in the morning and before I ate my lunch and dinner meals, (2) eating precisely the amount of carbohydrate grams I had been instructed to eat on a daily basis – and no more, (3) getting thirty minutes to an hour of exercise at least four times per week, and (4) making sure I took my medications as prescribed. It was non-negotiable. I didn't think about it. I didn't agonize over it or feel sorry for myself about it (very often). I just did it all. I didn't need a drill instructor.

I had the Diabetes Monster breathing down my neck.

By "just doing it" (as the advertisements suggest), it was infinitely easier on my psyche in those early months. After all, I had a paid position to attend to, laundry to do, groceries to buy, papers to grade, and a life to live. Just like always. Nobody could tell by looking at me that I was teetering on the brink of a physical and emotional meltdown. And when my job became permanent at the end of the semester, I got an opportunity to move to an apartment I liked much more, so there was all that to deal with. In other words, not going haywire was allowing me to feel like an ordinary person, which I, of course, was, no matter what my over-active brain cells were screaming.

Areas 1, 3, and 4 have remained a more or less absolute part of my life ever since. Issues related to what I eat have morphed somewhat from time to time, which I will discuss later in the section on food. But, since my diagnosis, I have gotten up every single morning and stuck my finger so I know my glucose reading. Like going in the bathroom to pee. It just has to be done. So I do it. And testing my blood glucose level remains the basis for my management system begun in boot camp.

I was originally issued a particular brand of glucometer, which worked fine, but I changed to another brand a couple of years later, when I discovered that the Freestyle Lite[iv] glucometer would make the necessary reading with the tiniest bit of blood imaginable. And the smaller the drop, the smaller the stick, and the less sore the fingers. The Freestyle Lite also beeps when the blood drop registers, lights up so it's easier to read, and has great big numbers, all of which I found appealing.

Regardless of which brand you choose, however, if you pay attention, it's not difficult to get a glucometer for free because companies are willing to give them away to lock in a permanent order for the particular test strips that go with their meter. You can find such offers in those free diabetes magazines at the doctor's office or you can look online, especially on the websites for the products you're interested in. The difference between the Freestyle Lite and the first meter I used was fairly radical and my fingers were immediately very grateful.

In the zippered kit holding the meter and the test strips that I carry everywhere I go is also the spring-loaded mechanism I use to stick whichever finger is drafted into use because it's no longer sore. The lance (as it's called) can be set to make the smallest prick you'll need to produce enough blood to register on the meter. To give you an idea of how little blood is required for the Freestyle Lite glucometer, I set the lance on "1" for the first few years and have only recently progressed to the setting "2". And that's after seven and a half years of testing.

The generalized instructions I received initially call for changing the lancet (the part that sticks the finger) every single time you want to test, the rationale being that, otherwise, the lancet will get dull, it will hurt more, and will be more prone to produce calloused fingertips. But I choose, instead, to replace the lancet before I go to bed, using a fresh lancet each day, but not with every stick. Since I'm on the go a lot and have to carry my kit, I want to limit the amount of necessities I must carry, especially now that it includes insulin, alcohol swabs, and so forth. And changing it daily doesn't seem to have created any extra problems for my poor little finger tips[v].

I was always concerned that during or after testing my glucose, I might get a blood spot on my clothing. So, not knowing what else to do, I developed the habit of licking my finger after the meter tells me my glucose level. I felt a little Neanderthal about it until I read recently (after seven years of doing it) that this is what most folks do. So there you have it, for what it's worth. Additionally, by and large, I prick my fingers on the sides by my fingernails rather than in the middle or on the very end because it hurts less.

Over time, I began testing more and more, which is the only way I can tell what my glucose level is. Sometimes, when my glucose is low, I may tremble or feel flushed, my scalp may tingle, and I may start to sweat or feel sleepy. But sometimes, I can be just as low without any of those symptoms. And, of equal concern, I can be high, even quite high, without any symptoms at all. So my only sure option is the meter.

During periods when my glucose seems uncharacteristically unpredictable, I might test as many as six or seven times per day. And just after I began using insulin, my levels were so out of control, I was testing ten or twelve times per day in an effort to manage them.

Some instructions suggest that we should take glucose readings right before we eat and again two hours after we're done eating, in the interest of staying carefully in a safe range (not below 70 and not above 180). But reality for me (and for others I have talked with) is that your BG (blood glucose) level can sometimes be inexplicable.

The first five years after my diagnosis, my fasting BG (first thing in the morning) was virtually always somewhere between 85 and 115. But if I was even a little under the weather or didn't sleep well or was going through some emotional upset, it might be 160. And there are a couple of other ways it can be high in the morning without any of those things going on: one being the Dawn Phenomenon (caused when your liver dumps glucose into your system as a response to the release of the hormones you need to get rocking in the morning) and the other being the Somogyi Effect (caused when your liver dumps glucose into your system as a response to your BG dipping too low in the night). Eating a Greek yogurt right before going to bed around 10 p.m. and then eating breakfast as soon as I get up at 6 a.m. seems to lessen the likelihood of these issues for me.

I often dealt with a high BG later in the day by taking a brisk two-mile walk or ducking into the gym to ride the stationary bike for a half hour. It was amazing to me how just running around the park for a while could take my BG from 185 to 90 in thirty minutes. But between the way I carefully regulated my food intake and my oral medications, it didn't happen a lot during those early years. And I thought I had it all figured out. Until my pancreas simply quit producing insulin so I could no longer manage my disease, that is, which I will cover later in the book.

Checking my BG before meals saved me from being "naughty" *many* times when I was considering foods that would have sent my glucose level even higher than it already was. And this brings us to the topic of food, which requires a section of its own.

---

[i] Some people diagnosed with diabetes while they're severely overweight discover that their body stabilizes when they lose enough pounds, but this isn't by a long shot the bulk of us.

[ii] See a very different story described in the Appendix to this book.

[iii] One of my favorite websites and a great one to begin with can be found at www.dlife.com. If you register there and include an email address, they will keep you posted about all sorts of helpful information in a user-friendly format. They also offer training webinars online about pertinent topics. But once you start looking for information on diabetes on Google, in no time at all, you'll be bombarded with other options.

[iv] I'm going to refer to brand names from time to time in this little book because it's information I wish I'd had when I was first diagnosed. Personal preference, needless to say, might dictate that you prefer a different brand of some product or food I might mention, but at least you'll be starting out with more information than I had. I have not received any encouragement or compensation for mentioning anything in this book.

[v] The Freestyle lancets I use, by the way, are 28 gauge sterilized stainless steel. Gauges run from 23 to 30. The lower the number, the bigger the hole will be and the more the pricks will hurt. Apparently, my skin isn't too thick, so I can use a lancet that makes a pretty small entry hole. Thank goodness.

Part 4

Eating to Live, Not Living to Eat

I once knew a man, who, when I asked him what he believed in, thought for a moment and replied, "I believe...food." I thought it was a very clever answer and I never forgot it. Whatever belief systems humans may have developed over time on this planet, we all certainly believe food. We can't live without it. We derive major pleasure from it. We create rituals around it and the sharing of it. We craft cultural traditions based on it. We grow it. We prepare it. We talk about it. We even take pictures of it to send out to our friends on our cell phones. We *believe* food.

When a newly diagnosed diabetic is introduced to the rigor of managing his or her food intake, it can feel as if we're being cut off permanently from the rest of the human race. We haven't committed a crime. But we're being punished. We still want to eat what others are eating. But we can't. Or at least we can't if we want to keep living. Yet we need to eat to live. It's complicated.

Our family and friends may be supportive. They may even feel sorry for us. And they may try to get us to "stick to our diets." But they don't have to forego the things we can no longer even think about, if we're smart. And it *hurts*. It's hard for them to get their brains around it. Just yesterday, we were *all* eating smothered chicken, mashed potatoes with gravy, corn on the cob, and hot biscuits, washing it down with big glasses of sweet tea and finishing it all off with apple pie *a la mode*. And one day later, they still *can*. But we can't. It's not their fault. They're not going to give it all up just because *we* have to. *We* don't want to give it all up and we *need* to.

So we tell ourselves we'll be careful tomorrow. Or that this is a birthday party after all (it would be *rude* not to partake). Or whatever comes to mind that allows us to make the decisions that can cost us our lives. Until we wind up in the hospital and then life goes on as usual for everybody else. But not for us. It's no wonder diabetics as a group are said to be the most depressed people in America.

During my Boot Camp stage, I was living alone, which probably made it easier for me to stick to my regimen. I only kept in the house what I could eat. And I kept a stash of appropriate food choices at the office. Lean Cuisines in the freezer in the faculty lounge. Nuts, dried figs, and chewy granola bars in my desk drawer. And Hershey's dark chocolate nuggets with almonds (at 5 grams of carb each) for when I just *had* to have a little treat. I never ate more than two and usually only one at a time – and *never* as a "snack." Which allowed me to have "dessert" without hurting myself. Did I want rice pudding or pecan pie instead? Sometimes, yes. But that would hurt me. The small bit of chocolate after a meal helped me to satisfy my need for a treat while not compromising my commitment to continue living a quality life.

When I went elsewhere, like a public event or a buffet, for example, I developed a practice of scanning the table first to see what I could have. Fried chicken? (Okay, but hidden carbs in the batter.) Green salad? (Okay, but not with heavy dressing.) Fresh green beans without the cream of mushroom soup added? (Yes!) Fruit cocktail in heavy syrup? (No!) And all the things I'd let myself have two bites of: potato salad, baked beans, cake with the icing scraped off. I found that if I let myself have two bites[i] of a few "bad" things, I was less likely to eat more than two bites. I learned to relish those bites, to really love and enjoy them. And, that way, I didn't wind up feeling like I was on the outside looking in. Denying myself entirely would have jacked up my self-pity and resentment about what others were eating (as if they were doing it to be mean). And the next thing you know,

I'd be standing behind a tree or in the hallway stuffing something forbidden into my mouth while I hoped no one was looking.

When the university would offer free strawberry shortcakes on a holiday, I'd stand in line for mine, eat two bites and throw the rest away. I don't belong to the "clean plate club" any more. I belong to the "I want to live to see another day of fun" club. And I still got my taste of the yummy.

Occasionally, I even get a pleasant surprise. I remember going to Junior's in Grand Central Station with my daughter for lunch one day the year after I was diagnosed.

"They have a low carb cheesecake here you might like to try," she informed me as we finished our burgers (mine without bun, hers loaded).

"Oh, I don't know..." I hedged, when I saw that it only had 4 grams of carb per serving. "I haven't had very good luck with low carb dishes being tasty."

I should have realized immediately that no cheesecake would ever survive on a New York City menu if it didn't rock, but I was still discouraged with my situation. Nevertheless, I ordered it and discovered a new Truth: there *are* people out there that know we exist. That cheesecake was *delicious*! I had a slice. My daughter had a slice. We took home a whole cheesecake when we finished. And we've made a habit of buying another one every time I'm in New York City since.

Sometimes, however, though my craving centers are going off like gang busters, I decide to leave whatever it is that set them off alone. I think about it. I want it. And I walk away. That's my trick. I don't tell myself no exactly. Because right at that moment, I don't want to hear it. But I just walk away with the thought that while it would be tasty, it would not be good for me. Ten minutes later, I've moved on.

Actually, this is a trick I learned how to use earlier in my life when I wanted to act on some impulse not in my best interests.

That instantaneous urge may feel *very powerful*, but ignored, often lessens fairly quickly – especially if you know perfectly well there *will* be consequences. The longer I agonize over the decision, the worse I know it is for me. Otherwise, I would just have done it. So why would I want to hurt myself? I've done that enough in my life.

This also works when I look at a menu. I'm partial to Reuben sandwiches, but they spike my glucose level. So when I see them on the menu, I might say to myself, "Ummm...that sounds so good." But then I consider how I'm going to feel later when I look at my glucometer and see a reading I know means I've done myself damage. And I choose something I like, but which won't have that effect. It's not as though the choice is between pumpkin pie and mud. I'm eating something I like, just not something I like that will *hurt* me.

Every time I win the struggle against an inadvisable urge, no matter what it is, I feel like a super hero, my own best friend, and the grown up I choose today to be. Not only does it get easier to walk away every time I do it, but the fear of the disease that I had initially *also* lessens, because *I* am in control. Ha! Take *that*, Diabetes Monster!

The minute I was diagnosed diabetic, shopping for groceries became an exercise in label-reading, which it has remained. It's astounding how many products are loaded with hidden carbs. A small bottle of catsup has 6 tablespoons of sugar in it besides the carbs from the tomato puree itself. (So imagine what the grams of carbohydrate are in white potato french fries, each one carrying a scoop of catsup!) Peanut butter[ii] only requires peanuts and salt, but virtually all the most popular brands have sugar added. And why do food companies put sugar in canned sweet peas?

Sugar is not the only hidden carbohydrate, however. If you read the labels on canned soups, for example, you'll find that some cans of Campbell's Chunky soup list only 15 grams of carb in each of the two servings the can holds. While other cans list twice that much or more. And notice that I said the can will tell you there are two servings in that can, so the carbs listed on the label relate to each serving, not the entire contents of the can[iii]. This is also something I learned to watch for in many other packaged food products. If I can only eat half of the product and still stay in my carb range, it might not be enough food to satisfy me, so I make a different choice.

It's all well and good, of course, to say you're going to avoid packaged foods entirely and cook everything you eat from fresh ingredients (as the magazines encourage us to do with succulent dishes presented in brilliantly colored photos). Some of us have the time, commitment, and expertise to do it. Or have somebody else who will do it for us. But there are several problems with this they rarely discuss at any great length in the articles.

One is that we don't all have the time. The pace of life in the U.S. is pretty frenetic for many people, what with jobs, kids, and housekeeping. I mean, everybody has to do their laundry at some point. And that's before we fold in the need to stay fit (non-negotiable for diabetics who want a quality life), as well as any social activities or volunteer work, organizational responsibilities, or church commitments. I have to pay my rent. I don't have time to fine chop spices I grow myself for my vegetarian chili. At the end of a long day, it feels like work. And what too many of us do about that is stop by the fast food joint on the way home and order a Value Meal with a side order of guilt.

Another, even trickier issue related to cooking tasty recipes is what diabetic nutritionists call "portion control."[iv] Whipping up a big skillet full of brown rice and veggies with chicken can make it *really* easy to put an extra scoop on the plate or in the bowl. And that extra scoop adds carbs, not to mention how it teaches your stomach to demand more food than is healthy – or necessary – for you. Everybody *else* is going back for seconds. Why can't you? After all (we tell ourselves), it has chicken in it and meat has no carbs at all.

One way I address this problem (still, after all these years) is that, if I'm at home and I'm preparing something myself, I actually measure the amount I want. I know exactly how much certain bowls hold, for example. But that doesn't necessarily prevent the "extra scoop." So if I want to eat a cup of cottage cheese (8 grams of carb and 26 grams of protein) with a cup of ripe, juicy cantaloupe (13 grams of carb), I break out the measuring cup. Every time. This is not just so I don't overdo it. I want to make sure that if I'm allowing myself 21 grams of carb for that part of my lunch or dinner, I get every delicious carb gram I'm allotted.

But let's say you make that big pot of whatever and manage not to eat extra scoops, another problem that arises is that, while leftovers are wonderfully convenient and, quite possibly, the best part of cooking from scratch, at some point, even if you have a family, you're likely to get so tired of facing brown rice and veggies with chicken day after day that you may never want to look at it again. It seemed like such a good idea at the time. But enough is enough.

I always think those beautiful color photos of food in magazines look irresistible, but the reality is simpler. I wouldn't necessarily like them all enough to make up for the amount of work put into them. I know prepared foods may cost more, but ingredients I have to buy for a given dish are going to cost, too – sometimes a lot – because I'll have to buy a whole product, can, or package of each ingredient for even a small amount of something I don't often use or won't use all of. My time is worth something, as well. And let's face it, not all of us have the skill or the patience to cook what we see in the photos. Besides, once you know how to read a label, it's not entirely an either/or proposition.

Food processing company executives are increasingly smelling the coffee. If we don't buy the stuff loaded with salt and full of chemical additives we can't even pronounce, they find a way to offer an alternative. Hormel Natural Choice Deli Sandwich Meats, for example, taste just as good as the other brands, are relatively reasonably priced if you don't use more than two slices on a sandwich, and conspicuously lack the chemicals and additives for which sandwich meat is infamous. But remember, no brand is above selling you garbage to make a dollar. So read the label. If you can get a similar product without the ingredients and carbs you don't want, opt for the similar product. If you don't like the flavor of the one that's better for your health, look for another. Go online and do a Google search. Or find something else to crave. Over time, it's interesting how our bodies shift to prefer the foods that do our body good. And then one day, you realize you have no desire for what you used to love.

Still, sometimes there are food products I want, whether they're good for me or not. Diet soda is one example that comes to mind. Most diet sodas have aspartame. And aspartame will kill you. A few years ago, I watched a good friend very nearly lose her life while one doctor after another tested her for every horrible disease and disorder known to medical science. At the end, she could barely stand. She was in agonizing pain 24/7. And she trembled like a leaf. After nearly a year of this, in desperation when the doctors just gave up, she went on the internet and discovered that her symptoms were consistent with aspartame poisoning. She quit drinking diet soda all day long and, almost immediately, knew she was on the right track. A few months later, you wouldn't have known she was ever ill.

Under these circumstances, having seen it for myself, and knowing full well that diet soda doesn't add a bit of nutrition to my diet, you might think that I would never lift a bottle or can of diet soda to my lips. But the fact is that every once in a while (like when I'm eating leftover pizza), I want one. My personal preference is IBC Diet Root Beer in the bottle. Tastes delicious. And doesn't have an aftertaste. But it does contain the artificial sweetener aspartame.

So I bought a six-pack at the grocery four months ago and I still have two left. Get the picture? Once in a blue moon, I'll order diet soda in a restaurant, but since few of them carry IBC Diet Root Beer, most of the time, I'm saved from myself. And the aspartame[v].

There's been a bit of discussion about other artificial sweeteners. And there's enough disagreement that I'm not going to try to outline it all. The jury is still definitely out on comparing them. But, in the end, it comes down to taste for most of us. At least as long as it isn't a proven killer, like aspartame. My personal preference is Splenda. But keep in mind, I don't use a lot of it and I don't use it myself to cook with. It says on the package that one little envelope is equal to two teaspoons of sugar. I used to put a couple of teaspoons of sugar in my coffee or my tea. So today, I use one envelope of Splenda. And it works for me.

I threw out my sugar when I was diagnosed, by the way, and simply don't use it any more – not even for cooking. I don't put it in or on anything. I don't "substitute" honey or fruit juice or stevia or anything else that's supposed to make things edible. I still cook, though I don't make desserts, and I don't feel as if I'm missing anything. I still have daily opportunities to enjoy something "sweet," if I want to, but for the most part, other than the dark chocolate nuggets with almonds or an occasional Pepperidge Farm Sausalito Cookie[vi], "treats" are "treats" to me. Not something I eat like it's a necessary food group.

We've been sold a bill of goods in our culture that life isn't worth living if we don't have a big refined sugar concoction after every meal and in between. It's addictive. It's expensive. It's not healthy for anybody. And in France, they eat salad for dessert, which doesn't appeal to me, but it's an example that "dessert" is an acquired taste that can be un-acquired.

Before you decide I'm an alien robot and can't relate to your struggle, though, I must tell you that I've always loved ice cream. My earliest memories of joy all involved ice cream. And I remember fondly (before I was diagnosed, of course) watching television while downing an entire pint of Ben and Jerry's New York Super Chunk Fudge ice cream – and I'm not just talking about once.

So I can't bring ice cream home in a container of any size. Not a quart or a pint. And certainly not anything bigger. If I do, once the plastic wrapper is removed, I will stand in front of the refrigerator with the freezer door open, scraping big spoonfuls off the top right out of the container and into my mouth. I just leave it at the store and don't kid myself.

On the other hand, I do allow myself every month or so on very special occasions, to stop at a Baskin-Robbins store and have one scoop of Jamoca Almond Fudge in a cup. It's 17 grams of carb. And I sit right there in the store and do everything but lick the cup out when I'm done.

I have also found a couple of other cold and creamy delights. Weight Watchers offers strawberry yogurt on a stick that I'm partial to, as well as chocolate covered toffee ice cream on a stick and both of them are only 12 grams of carb. They're not Ben and Jerry's, but they're tasty and if you only eat one, they're safe. My point (again) is that I am *not* suffering. If my favorites don't appeal to you, you can find your own. I'm just pointing you in the right direction and assuring you that there *is* a Promised Land.

After years of more or less always toeing the mark, I just automatically do a lot of things. Like only eating half of a small baked sweet potato and saving the other half for another meal. Or skipping carbs entirely in the meal so I can have some kind of real dessert afterwards. It sounds like cheating. But I originally got this idea the first time I talked to my diabetic nutritionist.

I listened to what she said about how many carbs I could eat each day, especially at mealtimes, and, ever cagey, asked, "Does it matter where the carbs come from?"

Her reply was music to my ears.

"Not within reason," she said.

And I was off to the races. Within the first few weeks, I had already, at least once or twice, eaten a Starbuck's salad with grilled chicken (and only the smallest touch of dressing) for lunch with a cup of coffee and...wait for it...a double chocolate chunk brownie or oatmeal cookie for dessert. At 41 and 40 grams of carb respectively, neither would destroy my BG if I was careful the rest of the day and didn't make a regular practice of it, especially if I worked out that day. After all, on most days, my lunch was a Lean Cuisine. This was not me being resistant to the need for vigilance where my blood glucose was concerned. It was me making sure that I didn't yell "Screw it!" one day and throw in the towel.

Making trades has become a common way of functioning for me, especially when I eat out. Ordering a cheeseburger at a decent restaurant, I have the server bring it without the bun and with a salad on the side instead of fries. Then, I beg five or six of my dinner partners' fries if I have one. Or order fries, eat ten or fifteen and send the rest away. I try to order salad dressing with the fewest hidden carbs (raspberry walnut vinaigrette[vii] being my favorite) and have it served on the side, using only the least possible amount to wet the greens and no more. If I want to have blue cheese dressing and a few croutons, I'll eat fewer fries. I avoid appetizers unless they're all protein (like shrimp cocktail or grilled oysters). I stay away from fried foods, by and large, because the batter is loaded with hidden carbs. I never touch the breadsticks or the crackers that come with the meal (or I only take two bites). I routinely push the rice pilaf around far more than I eat it. And it works.

I've even discovered a pizza I can have at my favorite pizzeria. I order an individual (8") combination pizza with thin, whole wheat crust and zesty sauce (meaning they leave out the sugar). I eat half of it at dinner and take home the other half for lunch the next day. Do I walk away from the table moaning about how full I am? No. But I walk away from the table after eating delicious pizza, carrying a box with delicious pizza for tomorrow. Not being able to have *everything* I want doesn't mean I'm "suffering." Remember?

When I was diagnosed diabetic, my A1C was 10.9. This is the calculation that tells the doctor how high the diabetic's BG averaged for the ninety days just prior to the test. I could explain how it's calculated, but it's not necessary to know and the information is easy to find elsewhere (like on the internet), if you really want to understand it. Suffice it to say that, if you take the A1C number times thirty, you get roughly the average BG level. So, when I was diagnosed, my average BG was probably running around 327, and I was already dealing with complications.

Six months later, what with watching my carbs, taking my medication, and doing regular exercise, my A1C was down to 5.8

or an average of 174. That wasn't awesome because the target area is between 80 and 120, though most doctors are not too horrified if it's a little higher. But it was a whole lot better than what it had been before and the blurred vision, constant thirst and 2 a.m. trips to the bathroom were a thing of the past.

YOUR LIFE ISN'T OVER

---

[i] This means standard size bites – on the smallish side – rather than mouthfuls masquerading as bites.

[ii] It should also be noted that homogenizing peanut butter so it doesn't separate from the oil in the jar before it's opened makes the protein hard to assimilate. If you want peanut butter that does your body good, you can try Smucker's old fashioned smooth or crunchy style peanut butter. You'll see that the oil has separated, so when you open it at home the first time, just take a sturdy knife and stir the peanut butter (all the way to the bottom) until it's thoroughly mixed, close the lid and refrigerate the jar. It won't separate again until it's all gone and you'll be getting excellent protein with no sugar added.

[iii] I made a big mistake a few times when I bought and ate something I thought was only a small carb splurge and then later realized that it supposedly had two or even three "servings" in the package – meaning that I had just eaten two days' worth of carbs all at once. There is apparently no standard for what constitutes a serving. So don't be caught off guard.

[iv] Unfortunately, the nutritionists' who talk about "portion control" and whoever chooses the recipes for those magazines are not always on the same wave length. I wish I had a nickel for every time I've looked longingly at a beautiful dish of food in a magazine for diabetics, wondering if I should break down and make it, only to discover that it has 45 grams of carb in ¾ of a cup. What would be the point of making something I could only have ¾ of a cup of?

[v] Aspartame doesn't just show up in diet soda either. So look out for this killer. Sometimes it's also added even when a product advertises itself as containing stevia or some other "natural" sweetener instead. But the aspartame will be

embedded in the list of ingredients, if you read them. There is a growing backlash against aspartame, however, which is why some products actually declare "No aspartame" on the label. They know.

[vi] Chocolate chip cookies with macadamia nuts that are the real deal and only have 17 grams of carbohydrate.

[vii] If you're eating at home, Newman's Own has a great one that's all natural, delicious, and all the profits go to charity.

Part 5

To Market, To Market

I've already mentioned a few products that you might find worth checking out, depending on how your taste buds operate. But in this part of the book, I'm going to list a few others that are staples at my house. These particular foods and products are not, by any means, the only things a diabetic can eat. And if you're lactose intolerant or allergic to nuts or under a doctor's orders not to eat fruit or whatever, just scan this part and move on. And you'll have to figure out what works best for you for yourself. But these are options for me, as well as many others. And I've discovered over time since I was diagnosed that the world is full of possibilities.

One woman I know told me that when her significant other was first diagnosed diabetic, he decided, in a panic, that the best way to avoid high glucose levels was simply to eat no carbs at all. This is *not* an option. Carbohydrates are to humans what gasoline is to cars. They fuel our bodies (including our brains). If we don't have enough carbs, our body will resort to eating our muscles for fuel. Which doesn't sound like something you would want to volunteer for.

At peak performance, the human body is a very efficient system. We largely take it for granted. And often treat it far worse than we treat our cars. It wouldn't occur to me not to maintain my car responsibly because I need it to work right. I don't want to get in it and have it refuse to start. I don't want to be on the highway and have my car cost me my life or send me to the hospital or even inconvenience my day. So, while I don't know a lot about how a motor works, I know enough to have it checked from time to time and I make sure the fluid levels are what they're supposed to be, that the tires are filled with the appropriate amount of air, and that I'm using the correct kind of gas. And I don't try to take it where it's not supposed to go. It's my car and it's my job to take care of it.

Technically, this is what medical professionals mean when they tell a diabetic: "each body is different" and "you'll figure it out." This can be daunting for the newly diagnosed, but even if the professional tells you to "do this" or "do that," the instruction may very well need to be tweaked in short order because they often don't know for sure how your particular body will react to the treatment. Sometimes they joke: "Well...that's why they say we 'practice' medicine. It's not an exact science." Which is not a great consolation to a person who's just been told they have a terminal illness.

For diabetics, food intake is just another aspect of our treatment. We must have carbohydrates to run our bodies and our brains. Knowing how different carbohydrates affect your particular body, though, is going to be important. And there's only one way to find out. So food intake is going to be a constant process of elimination (no pun intended) to determine what takes good care of you and what causes problems. And just to make it an adventure, your body won't always interface with a given food in exactly the same way. So one day, you may eat a certain amount or a certain food and have your glucose level stay low and on another day, the same amount or food will spike your BG.

The first bunch of times this happens it can be pretty unsettling. I used to go into a frantic tailspin because I thought that one high BG would take me down for the count, as it were. But that's not true. Still, you don't want it happening on a regular basis. And it's *you* who'll be going to the hospital or going blind or losing a foot, so *you're* the one that needs to pay attention. Ask a lot of questions. Read magazines for diabetics so you know what questions to ask. And test your glucose level regularly. It's on you.

I've learned, for example, that 1 cup of cooked Quaker Oats Old Fashioned oatmeal

(27 grams of carb) often spikes my BG. Shouldn't, but it does. Quaker Maple and Brown Sugar Instant Oatmeal, on the other hand, which I normally eat with one chopped date, a tablespoon of chopped walnuts, and a splash of soy milk (for a total of 39 grams of carb) doesn't. Go figure.

And while we're talking about oatmeal, if you try the instant oatmeal I just described, when you first look at the bowl, it won't look like enough food. But if you prepare it the way I do with a slice of Nature's Own 100% Whole Grain bread, toasted with butter (12 grams of carb) and a cup of coffee or tea, it's remarkably satisfying. Especially once you get used to not force-feeding yourself at every meal.

The bread I eat, by the way, is a good example of my own personal process. I've been eating whole grain bread since the 1970s – the heavier, the better. If I could differentiate the various grains in the bread, I loved it. But when I was diagnosed diabetic and realized that bread like that often has as much as 25 grams of carb per slice and that, because of that, I was only going to be able to eat half a sandwich at a sitting, I didn't know what to do. I was habituated to that heavy bread. I eat a lot of sandwiches. But a half a sandwich wasn't going to do it.

So I started reading bread labels until I found the bread I mentioned above. It's not as heavy as the kind I used to enjoy, but it's still whole grain, so it has more heft to it than regular whole wheat does. And it only has 12 grams of carb per slice. What I had done with my research was find a loaf of bread I liked that had few enough carbs that I could eat a whole sandwich. See how it works?

If you're like me, you've probably been eating the same things (and especially the same brands) for years. Without any thought. Products change every day, though. Literally. So there may be all kinds of products and foods out there that you would just love if you "have to" look for them.

Do I still prefer the seriously heavy bread? Yeah. Sometimes, when I know I'm going to be working late, I'll buy a turkey and Havarti cheese with cucumber sandwich (on heavy whole wheat) from Starbuck's (because we have one on our campus). I'll eat half of it for lunch (22 grams of carb) with half of a double chocolate chunk brownie (22 grams of carb). And with a cup of coffee, I'm good. Then, at my desk, working through dinner, I'll break out my remaining half a sandwich and half a brownie and love them all over again. I am *not* suffering.

If there are items you could eat, but have never tried, even if you think you're going to hate them, you might want to pick them up at least once to see for sure. I was offered Greek yogurt multiple times at a local organic foods store years ago and swore I didn't like it (for some reason). Today, I think I could live on it. Weird. So assume nothing. You never know.

Another thing I don't quite understand, but is definitely worth knowing about BGs and food is that if you eat more protein, carbs are less likely to spike. So if you're in the mood for a Cinnamon and Raisin English Muffin (with 29 grams of carb) for breakfast, rather than spreading it with cream cheese, put a slice of turkey and a slice of Swiss cheese or an egg on it and you're more likely to stay in range. This doesn't mean that eating a steak buys you the chance to down a gigantic loaded baked potato. But it adds a bit of wiggle room to your meal.

Having said all that, here are some other things that might help you get started on your own journey.

STAPLES

Vegetables – Vegetables are an important staple for the diabetic's diet, but even vegetables have to be carefully chosen. There are low carb vegetables, like green beans (7 grams of carb per cup) or broccoli (6 grams per cup) and then there are high carb vegetables, like peas (21 grams per cup) or corn (123 grams of carb per cup!). I'm not going to give you a long list because I don't know which vegetables you might want to consider and besides, the information is readily available on the internet, in carb counting booklets you can pick up at the grocery store, or just from reading labels. Remember to be careful to notice not just the amount of carbs, but the amount of food the calibration uses. A half cup of food is almost not enough to think about, unless you're mixing it with something else. On the other hand, two bites of buttered corn on the cob can taste like heaven, if you remember to stop at two.

I eat a big salad as a meal on a regular basis, mixing 2 cups of Dole Classic Romaine salad (6 grams of carb), half of a small avocado (6 grams), half of a small apple, chunked, or some blueberries (7 grams), grated cheddar cheese, 2 tablespoons of chopped walnuts; some cut up ham, leftover chicken, or deli turkey salad; and 1 tablespoon of Newman's Own Raspberry-Walnut Vinaigrette (5 grams).

That's a total of only 24 grams of carbohydrate for a big bowl of very tasty food. And it's balanced with protein, vitamins, minerals, fats, and fiber, and leaves me free to eat a Pepperidge Farm Sausalito Cookie for dessert.

Fruits – Fruits have a bad reputation, but as you can see above, not all that reputation is earned. It's true that, at 24 grams of carb, 8 ounces of orange juice is out of my league. But almost any kind of berries are fairly low. I buy small apples or only eat a half. If I buy canned fruit, it's always in 100% fruit juice (no syrup, no sugar, no artificial sweetener) – and I drain the juice. Melon is fairly low in grams of carb, but I have to watch watermelon because I want to eat too much. A cup of watermelon may only have 11 grams of carb, but most of us are only getting started with a cup of watermelon. Go get a measuring cup and see what I mean.

One thing about fruit, though, is that, if you're not eating a lot of refined sugar products in your diet, fruit does a great job of satisfying the yearning for something sweet and it's really good for you. You still have to count the carbs, but I have a bit of fruit with every meal: a small tangerine, six or seven dark cherries, or a half a cup of pineapple chunks, any of which only adds 10 grams of carb and all of which add juicy sweetness to my lunch or dinner, as well as a flavor burst to keep things from getting boring. Sometimes, just the addition of two dried dates (5 grams of carb each) or a fig (8 grams) can cap a meal deliciously.

Grains – I've already told you how I worked out my sliced bread problem, but cereal was quite another issue. It turns out cereal is the devil. Most of it has something like 40 grams of carbohydrate in one-half cup. I wouldn't dirty a bowl for that much. So I had to read a *lot* of labels before I decided that I had two choices: I could just leave cereal alone entirely or I could eat Cheerios. Not Honey Nut Cheerios or Multigrain Cheerios or whatever flavor of the month Cheerios comes out with. Just plain Cheerios with no sugar on top.

Regular Cheerios only has 20 grams of carb per cup, so on a day when I feel like cereal, I can eat a cup and a half of cheerios with a half a cup of fresh strawberries and a cup of unsweetened soy milk for a total of 39 grams of carb. And I'm a happy camper. The strawberries sweeten both the cereal and the soy milk, but it can't be berries that have been sweetened with sugar. Capiche?

Greek Yogurt – Greek yogurt is high in protein and comes with a wide range of different amounts of carbohydrate grams. More importantly to many of us, though, it comes in many, many flavors. I eat Greek yogurt at any time of the day, depending on what my needs are and the grams of carb I want. But be aware that some yogurt has aspartame, which I avoid because it's easy. Also be aware that a little cup of yogurt might have as few at 8 or as many as 36 grams of carbohydrate in it. So, clearly, you want to read the labels.

Some flavors sound fabulous at the store and then aren't when you get them home, but if that happens to you, don't jump to the conclusion that they're all bad. My favorites include, among others, Muller Greek Yogurt with berries or caramelized almonds (22 grams of carb); Chobani Greek Yogurt with apple, cinnamon, and oats (27 grams of carb); Dannon Light and Fit Caramel Macchiato Greek Yogurt (8 grams of carb); and decadent Chobani Greek Yogurt with ingredients you "flip" into the yogurt and stir before eating in flavor combinations you need to read to believe (27 grams of carb). But with such a wide range of carbs, you know you have to pay attention.

On a particular day, for example, I might eat a Greek yogurt with 22 grams of carb for breakfast paired with a whole wheat English muffin (another 22 grams of carb) spread with peanut butter or cream cheese. I often eat a decadent Chobani "flip" before bed so that my BG doesn't dip too low in the night. And if I "crash" after a workout (meaning my BG goes below 70), I might eat a Greek yogurt with only 8 grams of carb so it doesn't ruin my next meal.

The difference between Greek yogurt and other yogurt is that Greek yogurt is creamier than regular yogurt, as well as higher in protein. And I know people who don't like yogurt at all. But all I can say is yogurt is a really nice addition to my bag of tricks. And I once read somewhere that there's a culture in the Caucasus Mountains where the people routinely live for more than 100 years and are healthy to boot. I don't know if it's true, but it works for me.

ODDS AND ENDS

Salt – I'll be the first to admit that I don't pay a lot of attention to salt. I know that some, maybe even many, processed or packaged foods are loaded with it (although this is changing). And I do like salted nuts and occasional French fries or chips. But I'm careful elsewhere. I almost never salt food at the table. I read labels and reject the worst offenders. And I've learned how to severely limit my intake of nuts, fries, and chips (even when I'm alone). For example, if I want chips with a sandwich at home, I opt for seven or eight Deep River Original

Salted Kettle Cooked Potato Chips (with sea salt). I buy them in the 2-ounce package so they don't go stale. I don't eat more than 1/3 of the package (which runs about 11 grams of carb) and they're committed to producing a healthier product. So I feel okay about it[i].

But when doctors put people on no-salt or low-salt diets, it's often because we're already at increased risk for high blood pressure, among other things. And this has to do, as much as anything else, with how much we weigh and how much or how little exercise we get. So, if you don't like being on a no-salt or low salt diet, lose some weight (see Part 2 of this manual) and start getting a lot more exercise. It won't happen overnight, but you will eventually get to have some of the things you're missing back in your diet. The reason the medical professionals take us off the salt is to keep us alive because they think we won't lose weight and do exercise. So surprise 'em. It's an option.

Sugar-free Products – The sugar-free

products I've tried tasted nasty, by and large. I may just have been trying the wrong products. But I think they're selling that stuff to people that think it's good for them when, actually, if you read the label, you often find the product has more grams of carb in it than another product that actually contains sugar. Remember: *sugar isn't the only hidden carbohydrate.* So before you buy that bag of "sugar-free" whatever, read the label (don't scowl – you're going to have to do this a *lot*) and then go ahead and compare it to products that are not sugar-free. *Before* you buy. Otherwise, I'm guessing you're going to wind up with lots of half-eaten bags of this and that you won't eat. Ever. And probably shouldn't.

Additionally, while we're on the subject, you really don't have to settle for those little glucose tablets they tell you to buy in case your BG gets low. I carry Werther's Original Creamy Caramel Filled Candies myself. They chew up quickly and easily and I love the taste, which is nice because if my glucose is so low that I'm breaking out the candy, I might as well get a pleasant experience out of the deal. And, at 5 grams of carb each, two generally takes care of me[ii].

Guilty Pleasures – I already told you that, during my Diabetes Boot Camp period, I didn't allow myself much. Besides Hershey's Dark Chocolate Nuggets with Almonds after meals, I just kept my eyes on the road most of the time. But before bed, I used to have a cup of Celestial Seasonings Sleepytime Extra Tea (a chamomile blend with valerian root) to help me unwind after a long and often stressful day. And I would drink it with three or four ginger snaps. Murray Old Fashioned Ginger Snaps have 4 grams of carb apiece, so that gave me a little something to go to sleep on and it was an every night affair. Since I started taking insulin, bedtime requires a bit more. So Greek yogurt has taken over. But I still remember those ginger snaps fondly. And you might like them, too.

Another guilty pleasure I've found is

Cary's Sugar-Free Syrup (the only sugar-free product I recommend unequivocally). With 11 grams of carb in a quarter of a cup, poured over two slices of French toast with a pat of butter and two turkey sausage patties on the side, I can feel just like everybody else on a Sunday morning. IHOP's provides Cary's, by the way, if you ask for it, but of course, they don't carry much of anything diabetics can put it on. Ah, well. At least it's a move in the right direction.

---

[i] When I go on a road trip, by the way, I'll take a little bag of these so I'm not tempted to pick up something worse at a roadside convenience store. And I'm careful to count my carbs, so I won't eat the whole bag at once.

[ii] There's only been a few occasions in seven years that I've needed something faster acting than the Werther's and I drank 4 ounces of regular soda or apple juice in those cases.

Part 6

Hut! Two, Three, Four!

Even when I was a teenager, I was never particularly into sports. We had to go to gym class, of course, and in the high school I went to, they required us to take swimming for credit. So it isn't that I never did anything physical. I could run and even high jump impressively for our annual Presidential Fitness Test. But I didn't think of it as something you would do by choice.

I lucked out to some extent, I guess, being born into a family that was built pretty sturdy. But other than that, I didn't even watch sports on television as a rule. Just wasn't interested.

So when they told me working out would help me manage my diabetes, it was about as meaningful as telling me I should start wearing an aluminum foil hat. I had no context into which to put the idea. Couldn't imagine where to begin. And certainly wasn't interested.

When I would come across some article about a diabetic celebrity whose personal trainer shows up at his house every day for a two-hour workout, I just thought he was showing off. I couldn't have a trainer come put me through my paces at a home gymnasium that didn't exist. And I didn't really understand the point anyway.

I joined the gym at the university I work for because the diabetic educator said I should. I signed up for ten sessions with a student trainer at the gym because I had absolutely no idea what to do with all those machines. I went several times a week for a few months. I lost 48 pounds and felt a little zippier. But I still didn't get what it had to do with diabetes.

When a boxing trainer I met convinced me a woman my age could "get in shape," I just thought it would make me look better in my clothes. I didn't have anything against that, especially since the weight loss had left me sagging here and there. And besides, there's been a fitness culture in the United States ever since we started buying running shoes and bottled water. Not that many of us actually ran, you understand, but we had the outfit if we decided to try it.

I don't know what got into me when I went to the animal shelter and came home with a sixty pound dog. I certainly didn't do it to ensure I'd be more active, but that's exactly what happened.

I had to go to work every day and VooDoo had to stay inside. So he needed to go out and take care of his business like clockwork in the morning and he didn't like going alone. So I would go with him, walk around the property a few times, watch him run off into the woods for a minute, and we'd go back in the house. After a while, it turned into jogging a few times around the property. Then, it turned into jogging down the road a little ways. And by the time winter came, I was ready to put on a sweat suit and gloves and jog two miles before work. And then three. And then four.

The next thing you know, I had added a little weight training and I was turning into an exercise geek. But I still didn't see any connection between the exercise and the diabetes.

By the time I won a 5K medal in my age range at a competition, though, I had noticed that if my glucose level was high, exercise would bring it down. Now *this*, I could work with. Especially since food and my emotions sometimes act on my glucose level in ways I can't predict. Or maybe I could have predicted, but didn't want to. So having an option in my bag of tricks for when I need it is a fall back plan I have appreciated greatly on occasion.

I normally do my exercise close enough to breakfast that I don't dip too low no matter how hard I work out, but in the summer, I have the option of going to the gym a little later. So I check my glucose level before I go and if it's below 165 or so, I eat a low carb Greek yogurt (8 grams of carb) or drink a WonderSlim pudding/shake[i] (7 grams of carb) on my way out the door and I'm fine.

Occasionally, if I finish exercising well before lunch, I might eat the low carb yogurt or drink the shake right *after* my work out. It keeps me from dipping too low, but doesn't jeopardize my being able to eat a full lunch when the time comes. My favorite shake flavors, by the way, are strawberry, mocha, and, of course, chocolate cream, but there are others. And they call it a pudding/shake because it comes in a packet and only requires ice water and a brisk shaking in a plastic Blender Bottle I bought when I bought my first box of packets. At $1.85 per packet, I wouldn't want to use these too often, but once in a while, it's just what the doctor ordered. Of course, the low carb Greek yogurt will accomplish the same thing, but the cold frothy sweetness of the shake is a very satisfying alternative[ii].

Eventually, I began to notice another excellent side effect of physical activity where managing my diabetes is concerned. If I'm physically active on a regular basis (at least four or five times per week, let's say), my glucose level actually stays lower than if I'm not. Apparently, exercise raises the Basal Metabolic Rate (the rate at which the body burns fuel). This is sort of like revving an engine. And the beautiful part is that, if I rev my engine four or five times a week, it keeps burning calories at the same rate even when I'm *not* revving it. This means I can eat more (and take less insulin) without my glucose being high. How cool is *that*?

More importantly, because of this, I'm less likely to develop complications. I'll burn fat. I'll develop muscles. And strong muscles help develop strong bones. Everything in the body is connected to everything else and exercise makes the whole system work better – even the brain.

Exercise lowers blood pressure, raises endorphins (the hormones that make us feel good), and because the heart is a muscle, it strengthens the heart. When I'm revving my body's engine, my heart is pumping more blood more quickly, so my body is able to get more oxygen and get rid of toxins more efficiently and at a higher rate.

In addition, diabetics tend to have problems with sluggish circulation and high cholesterol, both of which are also addressed by exercise. And on top of everything else, people that exercise routinely – whether diabetic or not – exude health. Their eyes shine, their hair shines, and there's a spring in their step. They tend to meet other people who exercise routinely. And let's be honest, active people just have a lot of fun.

Currently, my exercise rules are (1) never go two days in a row without doing some form of exercise, (2) switch up the activities so I won't get bored, and (3) have fun. Sometimes, I go over to the park and spend an hour speed walking and jogging around the running path. It's surrounded by trees and there's a pond with ducks and plenty of folks to speak to. Sometimes, when it rains, I use a DVD that guides me through a forty-five minute aerobic workout in front of my flat screen[iii]. Sometimes, I go spend an hour at the gym using the Ab Crunch and Back Extension machines, followed by pedaling a fast-paced five miles on the stationary bike[iv]. Some people watch television or listen to music or books while on the bike, but it slows me down when I do that, so I just think or meditate or pray.

Sometimes on a Saturday morning when the Farmer's Market and Art Fair is going on downtown and the weather's nice, I put on my shorts and running shoes and hustle the two miles down there, poke around a bit, grab a cup of cappuccino, and hustle the two miles back. It's fun. I get to see some of my friends. And I carry a lightweight bag on my back in case I find something I want to take home.

Lately, I've been toying with the idea of taking dancing lessons. I've always loved watching other people swing dance or jitterbug. And who doesn't love a masterfully executed tango? But I don't know how. The local ballroom dancing school keeps running an introductory offer in the newspaper and if I can find a partner who's willing to take the plunge, I think this has the potential to be a great exercise option I'll really enjoy. It'll burn carbs, it'll work my heart, it'll fine tune my sense of balance (which people of a certain age...*ahem*!) struggle with, and the next time I go to a dance, I'll be able to show off my moves.

Speaking of older bodies, by the way, my knees have started to act up a bit lately when I run, which is why I often just walk fast now rather than jog or I intersperse the two. But either seems to do the job and I still get my exercise. My point is that I originally started without much expectation related to what I was actually capable of. So I began slowly and worked my way up to the level of exercise I can now enjoy. And when things change, I change with it. Because that's always an option. But "exercise" is not all I do to stay fit.

For example, I always take the stairs instead of the elevator at work, where my office is on the third floor and my principle classroom is on the first. If I need to go across the campus to the library or the Center for Faculty Excellence, I walk. Fast. And sometimes I walk the mile and a half to work from where I live. If I go to an outdoor mall to visit a number of stores, I park in the corner of the parking lot, walk to do my shopping, and then walk back to my car. I'm even one of those people who walks around while they talk on the phone. In other words, I look for opportunities to build activity into my daily life.

Does that mean I never sit? Hardly. I spend a ridiculous amount time at a computer. I love to read. I watch Netflix. And I love to chat with my friends over coffee or a meal for hours. Which is all the more reason to exercise so that I can do all those things and have my glucose level unaffected. *wink*

ⁱ Available from www.wonderslim.com

ⁱⁱ Do avoid the ones that have aspartame as an artificial sweetener, though. They make the product available with or without it. Unfortunately, the kind without it has corn syrup solids instead, which are also touted as very bad for the body. But no more of these than I drink, I choose the corn syrup over the aspartame.

ⁱⁱⁱ My favorite one is Leslie Sansone's Walk Away the Pounds Ultimate Collection, which gives me the option to do one, two, three, or four mile challenges depending on how much time I have. It also comes with a stretchy resistance band she uses for part of the routine, but a couple of discs in my neck are herniated, so I get on the floor and do leg lifts or break out the five pound weights when that's going on.

^{iv} Once I started taking insulin, I had to be more careful when I went to the gym because my glucose level could actually drop so low that I couldn't continue my workout. One of the staff members suggested that I do my machine work first and the bike riding second and my glucose level wouldn't drop until I was ready to go home anyway. Any aerobic activity (exercise that makes the heart beat faster) pushes the glucose level down at a quicker rate than other forms of exercise.

Part 7

The Tool Kit

Everybody that has lived for more than ten years has probably, at least once, slammed a nail into a wall, a floor, or some other surface with the heel of a shoe. It doesn't necessarily work really well. And it's definitely not good for the shoe. But we do it.

On the other hand, most folks who've been living on their own for awhile (myself included) have a few tools at home to accomplish various tasks and the first one we buy, as a rule, is a hammer. Because it gets the job done *right*. Hanging a picture. Repairing a step. Putting up a shelf. You never know what you might want to do around the house, but a hammer, at least, plus a pair of pliers, a couple of screw drivers, and a wrench or two are pretty basic to the average household tool kit.

There are a set of tools I use to manage my diabetes, as well. They don't fit in a box under the kitchen sink. But it amazes me sometimes how well they take care of specific issues that have come up for me in the past seven years. You may not choose to use one or more of them for whatever reason. There are lots of people who don't see a need for a hammer when they already have a perfectly good shoe on their foot. But for the rest of us, there are options.

You may not initially realize how important some of these are to those of us with diabetes. You may be using some of them already without being aware of how crucial they are for you now. But just in case you've never tried a particular tool, I want to tell you what they do for me. Then, you can make up your own mind.

Sleep – I used to be a serious night owl back when I was young. And even when I was in grad school as a middle-aged woman, I burnt the candle at both ends *and* the middle. I was never one of those folks that fall asleep on the couch in front of a television. I was one of those folks with two speeds: on and off. And I spent a fair amount of time on. Particularly if I was writing. Which I do a lot.

Then came diabetes. I could still stay up, but if I did, when I woke up in the morning, I was liable to have a blood glucose level higher than normal and I felt wilted all day long. Still, I told myself that we gotta do what we gotta do and I just kept pushing. I'd throw down a little extra coffee, which then, of course, would make me feel artificially amped and make it that much easier for me to stay awake again. I wasn't going to be one of those old people that went to bed at ten – not *me*!

I'm fairly certain that one of the reasons I didn't want to go to bed before 11:30 or 12 was that I was dragging home from work at 7:00 or 8:00, sometimes later. By choice. I spent a lot of my day at work either teaching in a classroom or working one on one with students. Which meant that I had paperwork to do after everyone else left. And I also spent evenings at the campus – often – attending various student events to which I was readily invited. I liked being one of the popular teachers and I liked the mentoring I got to do after hours.

And to be honest, I kept it just like that until I got on insulin. It was like driving a nail with a shoe, but I liked to brag about how much I got done in a day and there was nothing else for it. But when insulin came into my life because my pancreas was no longer producing enough insulin to manage, I began to get serious. Or at least my diabetes did. If I didn't get to bed by close to 10:00 every night, my glucose didn't seem to want to hear about all the *good* stuff I was doing to keep it low. It ignored my efforts until I quit bucking and just went to bed.

Once I accepted coming home from work about 6:00 and going to bed at night by 10 or 10:30, I not only felt more relaxed in general, more even tempered, and less exhausted (which often presented itself as a form of depression), but my glucometer rewarded me with readings I knew I could live with – literally. I thought I wouldn't get enough done. I thought my students would forget who I am. I thought I would feel like I was wasting time at home in the evenings. I thought I would lay awake in bed for hours every night. None of which turned out to be true. And soon, I felt so much better, I couldn't imagine why it took me so long to figure it out.

Water – I knew for decades before I was diagnosed that the human body is 70% water. People that think sweating is the best way to lose weight don't realize that you have to replace the water you sweat in order to stay alive. And when the body holds onto water inappropriately, something else is badly out of balance and needs medical intervention. The water itself is not the problem.

Water is the way we cleanse our cells of toxins and move those toxins out of the body in urine, sweat, or tears. Not drinking plenty of water means the cleansing won't go on the way it needs to and our body gets sludgy with stuff we don't want to hold onto, even if we *don't* have diabetes to think about. This is why some people's urine is so dark. That dark color can be an indication that the water they **are** drinking is trying its best to do double-duty and carry all the toxins out of the system, but if we're drinking plenty of water, urine will be clear. In fact, the body needs water so badly that if we're not getting enough of it, we'll actually feel hungry, which makes us want to eat food when the body is really begging for water.

Even though I know all this, however, and do try to take in more water than some do, I often seem to get too busy to fill my water bottle. Or forget to drink the water even when it's full. Or drink the water and don't refill the bottle, as if one bottle is enough for a whole work day. I wouldn't drive my car without water in the radiator, but I will go all day often without so much as a sip of water myself.

A friend of mine brings four bottles of water to work every morning and makes sure they're empty by night. But I read somewhere that bottled water doesn't have to be monitored for purity like tap water does and that the plastic in the bottles can carry unhealthy chemicals. Not to mention that we're well into the process of covering the Earth with water bottles that don't biodegrade. And worse, bottled water is *way* more expensive than getting it out of the tap and filtering it yourself.

So I bought a bottle that's supposed to be made of chemical-free plastic and I refill it. But nothing can get the water out of the bottle and into my body but me.

Supplements – Before I list what I take in the way of supplements, I need to make clear that I'm not a doctor and I'm in no way suggesting that you take an over-the-counter substance instead of taking something a medical doctor has prescribed for you. I'm not an expert. When I scan the shelves and shelves of supplements in a store, I am invariably dumbstruck at the number and range of them all. And I've been taking some supplements for a very long time which have nothing per se to do with my diabetes.

However, I have become exposed to some information over the past seven years that has led me to decide to take several specific substances to assist in the treatment of my condition. I still take the drugs I'm prescribed (which I'm not going to go into because I don't want thousands of doctors to write me angry letters because their patients want to argue with them about why they are or are *not* getting exactly what I'm getting). Each body is different and every diabetic should listen to their doctor because he or she is trained to be responsible for prescribing their treatment.

Further, if you read the label on a supplement bottle, you'll find it makes a great point of saying that there is no conclusive scientific evidence that the supplement being bought is worth anything at all. Based on that, anything we spend is a waste. But I have shown my list to my endocrinologist (who I happen to think is brilliant) and he signed off on it. He didn't prescribe it, you understand. But he didn't tell me to stop taking any of it either.

If you know how to use the internet, I strongly recommend that you read up on these supplements yourself so you can decide which ones you might like to consider. They are not intended to take the place of medication or a doctor's care. I am not advising you to take them or even suggesting they will help you. I am simply telling you that, among all the supplements I take, I take three just because I'm diabetic and there is some indication they may help to manage glucose level in the blood. And that's good enough for me.

The first is R-Alpha Lipoic Acid[i], which I've read is often prescribed by doctors in Europe as soon as a patient is diagnosed either diabetic or pre-diabetic. I started taking this when my diabetes became unmanageable without insulin and I was beginning to develop what might have been neuropathy in my feet. Neuropathy is nerve damage and one of the early signs is tingling. I started feeling "something" after I went jogging and when I read up on the issue, I discovered that some research has suggested that R-Alpha Lipoic Acid can help to address this. I take 300 mg in the morning (with breakfast) and 300 more in the evening (with dinner) and I no longer feel the tingling. In all fairness, I started taking the insulin about the same time as I started taking the R-ALA, so maybe it was all the insulin. But I keep taking the R-ALA anyway.

The second supplement I take just because I'm diabetic is Potassium Gluconate (550 mg with breakfast). And the third is Chromium Picolinate (200 mcg with breakfast). And I don't have anything to say about either one of those except that I take them.

Meditation – I first became aware of meditation back in the 1970s when they introduced it into programs to rehabilitate people in prison. The results were pretty interesting in terms of how it changed people's attitudes and behaviors in a setting that could only be described as *very* stressful. But I never really embraced it personally at that time or ever, to speak of, until I became diabetic. There are lots of styles of meditation. Some fairly complicated and some so simple as to look more like strolling on a path. The bottom line is that any meditative practice that calms the body and the spirit can be helpful to diabetics.

I found out pretty quickly after I was diagnosed that getting angry would spike my blood glucose. But I wasn't getting angry too often during that time of my life. And when I did get angry, my glucose reading was the *last* thing I was thinking about.

But when I went on insulin, it seemed as if my body chemistry became super sensitive. Maybe it had nothing to do with the insulin. Maybe it had to do with the fact of my disease progressing so that my pancreas couldn't help me at all. I don't know. But whatever it was, if I got even a *little* bit hyped, my glucose level would go through the roof. One minute I'd be at 140 and a few minutes later, mid-argument, I'd be at 185 or higher, even *much* higher.

Of greatest concern to me those first couple of months on insulin was the fact that, because I tend to be pretty dramatic when I teach, amping up in a lecture was enough to send my glucose high. And that's what I do for a living. I was at a loss. There was nothing online about this. And the more I worried about it, the worse (and more predictable) it became.

Finally, I said to myself, "Well, I *have* to lecture. So I'll just do the best I can to deal with everything in my life right now. And worry about this later." I started breathing deeply with long, slow exhales on the way down the stairs to my classroom and, I swear to you, the spikes during my lectures stopped.

It still happens occasionally in situations like that, but not very often, and I just chalk it up to excitement. It might not happen to you, but when it happens to me, I use a breathing exercise and focus on soothing myself[ii].

This is basically what meditation does. Some people practice meditation for twenty minutes twice each day using fairly formal rituals. Others just take one-minute vacations in their minds while sitting at their desk at work. Sometimes, I like to focus on nature while I walk around the park, not thinking, not planning, just observing.

Sometimes, I lie down or sit quietly with my eyes closed and listen to a guided meditation (sometimes called a visualization). A voice on a cd or a YouTube video will take me on a little journey to let go of everything but the voice for five or ten minutes. And by the time it's over, I'm so still inside, I feel like a guru. I can't explain it, but it feels really good. You might like it, too.

Massage – I've always loved serious professional massages. I just couldn't usually afford them. Besides, I considered them something rich people do because they can. Just a guilty pleasure. And not for the rest of us. Then during a particularly stressful few months a year or so ago, I discovered that my chiropractor has a masseuse that works in his office and that I qualify for therapeutic massages when I go in for my adjustments.

I learned to value chiropractic adjustment when I was pregnant with my first child decades ago and I am a firm believer that when my spine is straight, my body in general works better. I don't know a lot about it, but it seems logical to me that since all the nerves in the body are connected to those that pass through the spine to reach the brain, it only stands to reason that a vertebra not in proper alignment would affect the whole system.

Not to mention the fact that once you know you don't have to be in pain, you want to avoid it. Right?

In any case, I now get massages when I get my spine adjusted and, besides the obvious benefits, I've noticed that for a period of at least 24 hours after my visits, my glucose stays so low, I have to take less insulin so I won't bottom out. I don't think there's any research on this, but I'm enjoying it anyway. And anything natural that reduces my glucose level *has* to be good for my body.

Therapy – I know there are a lot of people in the United States who think only raving lunatics need counseling. Which honestly, makes about as much sense as thinking you don't need a doctor unless a bone is broken. The reality is that few of us come through life unscathed. Whether it's childhood issues or time spent in a war zone or grief due to one or more losses or just needing to sort life out, *anyone* can get something from talking to a professional.

Some of us don't want to think about things that bring up pain. Which means that the pain stays down there inside us forever. We bury it and cover it with concrete and then disconnect our brains and tell ourselves we're not feeling anything. But we are. We just don't know it consciously. Not feeling pain that's supposed to be felt can kill you. Feeling the pain is the way to healing. Having to break up the concrete so we can let the pain out so we can quit feeling it can be scary, but I promise you that, with the right professional, it'll be worth it.

Finding a good therapist is just like finding a good mechanic to work on your car or a good hairdresser to cut your hair or a good anything else. You have to find someone you trust. You ask around. You try them out. And if the fit isn't good, you keep on moving until you find someone you feel okay with.

So what does this have to do with diabetes? I told you I was going to tell you about the tools in my tool kit. And going to a counselor is one of them. I have friends I talk with, but I don't ask them to fix my car or cut my hair and I don't expect them to be a professional counselor either. We might support each other in a lot of ways. We might comfort each other or give each other advice. But talking to a professional means I can say anything and it will stay in that room. It won't come up later unexpectedly and create an odd situation. It won't hurt anybody's feelings. And it's absolutely confidential. So, I can do a certain level of healing work with a professional that I can't do with anyone else. Doing that work has helped me become more comfortable in a troubled world and better able to meet the challenges of my life – including diabetes. Which can really be a stressor at times.

Artificial Calmatives – You might notice I don't mention a glass of wine with my dinner or a brandy before bed. I don't mention taking a drug to help me sleep or something to calm my nerves. I've learned to live without artificial calmatives other than the occasional cup of Sleepytime Extra Tea I mentioned earlier in the book. I'm not saying you shouldn't use them, though you might want to ask your doctor about that. And I'm sure that some diabetics find themselves wanting to medicate their feelings because of the stress of having the disease. But the tool kit I use to manage my condition doesn't contain anything of this nature and I seem to be doing fine.

---

[i] I compared the information and price on a number of brands of this supplement and have chosen to take Dr. Danielle's R-Alpha Lipoic Acid (300 mg capsules) because it's all natural and non-synthetic. Apparently, the synthetic ALA doesn't assimilate into the body as well as the natural ALA does. If the R doesn't appear in front of the word Alpha on the label, it's synthetic.

[ii] When we breathe in deeply through the nose and then exhale through the mouth until we empty our lungs completely – which we often don't do – it slows down the heart. Which slows down our mind. Which calms our body. Which can help to lower our glucose level. Nice, huh?

Part 8
Takin' My Best Shot

For whatever reason, the first question most people – diabetic or not – ask me is whether I'm Type 1 or Type 2. I don't think, by and large, they even necessarily know the difference. But the look on their faces when I announce my condition is a low grade of shock, followed shortly by sympathy. And I don't think they know what to say.

They've heard the terms "Type 1" and "Type 2," so they bring it up as a way to connect. Which is fine. I guess it's better than what they're probably thinking: some version of how glad they are it's me instead of them.

In any case, I don't assume from their question they have any idea what they're asking. And, regardless, I'm not really either one.

When I was diagnosed in February of 2008, the assumption was that I was Type 2. Type 1 diabetes typically makes itself known early in the life of the one who has it. Age fourteen is the average, more or less, but it can show up much earlier. It's marked by a lack of insulin being produced by the pancreas, so the administration of insulin as a medication is necessary immediately.

Type 2, on the other hand, usually develops in the late forties or after and does not necessarily ever require insulin at all, if the patient is able to manage their glucose level using diet, exercise, and oral medication. In fact, as I mentioned earlier in this book, if the diabetic is severely overweight when they're diagnosed and they lose sufficient weight, they may actually reverse their condition. It's not fool-proof, but it happens often enough that it's offered readily as a possibility when they're diagnosed.

I was 62 years old when I was diagnosed, but I was only about 30 pounds overweight and losing even 48 pounds didn't change anything. Diabetes doesn't run in my family and I was overall pretty healthy except for this startling news. I ate a healthy diet and lived a relatively active lifestyle, so even the medical professionals I saw seemed a little flummoxed at my condition. But there was no getting around it. I was diabetic.

For the first five years, I remained a diabetes "poster child" according to my doctor. I ran, did aerobics, and worked out with weights. I counted every gram of carbohydrate I put in my mouth. And I took my oral medications as prescribed without fail. I read articles and books on diabetes. I visited websites. I tested my glucose level multiple times a day. And my A1Cs (the blood test that tells what your average glucose level has been for the past ninety days) indicated that I was doing well.

Then, in year six, it seemed that nothing worked. My primary physician upped my medication. I tried to be more rigorous with my exercise. And I couldn't have eaten less without starving. Still, my glucose levels were often above 200, even right after I ran. I felt like a failure. And I thought I must surely be in some kind of downward spiral that could only wind up killing me. Depression hit like a brick and stayed with me. I didn't know what to think and I didn't know what to do. And I started to feel physically ill. I didn't realize it yet, but my next A1C was going to be 10.4, very nearly as high as it was when I was first diagnosed, indicating that my average glucose level, despite all my efforts to manage it, was running above 300.

When I finally walked into the endocrinologist's office, he took one look at me and said, "You don't look like a diabetic. Have you ever heard of Latent Auto-immune Deficiency in Adults? They call it LADA for short."

I assured him I had not, although I vaguely remembered my primary physician mentioning it in passing at one point. The next day, when I did my homework on it, I realized that I fit the profile precisely. Diabetes doesn't run in my family. I wasn't wildly overweight. But I developed diabetes anyway. It was manageable for about five years and then it wasn't, at which point insulin became necessary. So they call it Type 1.5.

The endocrinologist explained that they think LADA may result from the pancreas being damaged in some way. I recalled being extremely ill and in violent pain for a month a couple of years before my diagnosis. Ultimately, my gall bladder was removed and the symptoms stopped. But the endocrinologist suggested that I might well have had pancreatitis at the same time and it just wasn't identified.

"That can *kill* you, you know," he said pointedly.

"You mean I should stop feeling sorry for myself for being diabetic," I responded, "and dance in the streets because I'm alive?"

He nodded.

"I'll bet your pancreas has stopped producing the insulin you need," he went on, "so you don't have anything to manage. That's why your glucose levels have been so high. You need to take insulin now."

My stomach sank and my breath stopped. *Insulin?* The entire time since I'd been diagnosed, I had dreaded the day that I might hear that word. I had no idea when that development might occur or why. I just knew it was possible and I hated the thought. Every time I saw a magazine ad with some smiling person saying, "I was afraid of insulin, but now I love it," I would flip the page like it was in a foreign language. I didn't want to hear that. I couldn't imagine taking shots and still smiling. I didn't believe the ads.

"Are you needle shy?" the endocrinologist asked me.

"Would it make any *difference*?" I snapped back at him in despair.

But before I left the office, I had administered my first dose of insulin.

It went far better than I feared. Rather than the syringe I expected, the nurse practitioner brought in what looked like a magic marker and pulled off the cap. She showed me how to screw a very short and hair-thin needle onto one end of the pre-filled pen, then turn a dial to choose the dosage, pinch the flesh of my stomach and administer the medication. I barely felt it. In fact, it hurt less than pricking my finger to test for my glucose level. I was incredulous. *This* is what I had dreaded so badly? *This* is what had terrified me so much?

As I walked out of his office with a little brown bag of supplies, including insulin and orders to pick up more at my neighborhood Walgreen's, I felt surreal. My instructions were to take Lantus (a slow-acting insulin) once a day in the morning when I woke up and then Humalog (a fast-acting insulin) before each meal, the amount to be determined by how high my glucose was and what I was about to eat.

Walking to my car, I remembered how shell shocked I had been when I was first diagnosed six years before and how I eventually got the hang of it all. I remembered how I had survived the early months by just doing exactly what I was told to do exactly as I was told to do it. And I went into overdrive, breezing right past my panic and into the new regimen.

Still, rather than just thinking of the insulin as another form of medicine, I somehow got it in my mind that it was a thin string connecting me to life and that if it broke (because I couldn't get it), I would begin dying on the spot. It was summer and I didn't have to be in any classrooms, so my every waking moment soon filled with thoughts of insulin and how fragile I felt because of my disease.

Since the endocrinologist didn't yet know how little insulin my pancreas was producing or exactly how much insulin I needed to take, he started by suggesting a particular amount of Lantus and a sliding scale for Humalog and I was off to the races. Eight days later, I had gained eleven pounds. With the oral medication I was still on, the dosage of Lantus was too high and I was having to eat every two hours to keep my glucose from going so low that I might pass out. I was frantic. So I called and asked what I should do. I had already gone from 122 to 133. I had already outgrown all my clothes. And I had visions of soon being fat as a pig.

It was suggested that I try various combinations of amounts and we ultimately settled on taking me off the oral medication entirely and my taking an amount of Lantus less than 2/3 of my original dose. I continued to gain weight for a couple more weeks and then leveled off at 140, still appropriate for my height and putting me in a size 8 rather than the size 4 clothing I had been wearing for five years. Soon, I eased into my comfortable new routine.

The weight gain was obviously radical. I was haunting Goodwill in an effort not to invest in an all new wardrobe until I was sure my weight had stabilized. But, despite how much I liked being a clothes horse, I was secretly delighted. At 122, I was adolescent thin, but I didn't look really healthy. At my age and that weight, my face was a little haggard. I didn't have an ounce of fat, but I didn't have the figure I had always enjoyed having either. I actually loved being a new juicier me, as long as I didn't gain any more weight. That was a year ago and I'm still a size 8, but I have to work at it a bit.

The reason is that insulin gives you some options. It dawned on me, for example, at some point during the first week I was on it that I could now have Raisin Bran, my favorite cereal of all time, which I had left alone since my diagnosis because raisins are high in carbs. With insulin to balance it out, though, I could now have a bowl of the previously forbidden cereal and my glucose would still stay low. The trouble was that if I didn't work off the additional carbs, I would blow up like a balloon. Needless to say, I soon decided to leave the Raisin Bran at the grocery store and return, more or less, to the diet I was on before.

By my second week on insulin, I began to feel an emotional shift. The relief of discovering there was a specific reason why I couldn't manage my glucose level – and that I could do something about it – receded. Instead, I was left feeling a darkness that moved in and arm-wrestled the other feeling I was drowning in: being overwhelmed. And the tremor that sometimes shows up when I'm excited or under stress started appearing whenever it was time to take my insulin. Then, the more nervous I became about administering the medication, the worse the tremor got. And by the time I went in to see Debbie, my diabetic nurse educator, for a training session on insulin, I was no longer smiling at all.

"How's it going?" she asked me tentatively, watching my face for signals.

"Uh...it's okay..." I offered, not very convincingly. "But I'm worried about the fact that I've started trembling every time I need to take a shot. I wasn't doing that at first. And now that it's happening, the shots hurt a little bit and sometimes they bruise because my hand makes the needle shake after it's in the skin."

She made a couple of suggestions that sounded helpful and then asked quietly, "What thoughts have you been having this week that you didn't have last week?"

I claimed I didn't know, but then remembered, "This is going to be for the rest of my life..."

My voice dropped. My eyes went to the floor and would have welled with tears if I had let them. When I looked back at her, I knew my face was showing what I couldn't possibly say out loud: "Nobody can fix this or take this away. How can I do this forever..?"

"I was waiting for that," Debbie said with obvious relief. She needed me to put it on the table so we could talk about it.

I'm guessing I was going through a fairly typical process. I was somewhat numb the first week from the shock of this new development. But as the realization set in that I was now absolutely dependent on a medication that has to be injected one way or the other, the numbness had passed and low-grade terror had taken over. What if I ran out of insulin and couldn't get more? What if I lost my health insurance? What if my tremor got worse with age and I couldn't administer my own insulin? What if I needed someone else to take care of me and nobody was there?

Debbie had seen it all before. She loaded me down with so many brightly-colored materials on insulin-dependent diabetes, I needed a canvas bag to carry them home. She reminded me of how I had been frightened six years before when I was first diagnosed, but I eventually learned to handle both the fear and my diabetes. By the time I left, I felt able to meet the challenge. And the inexplicable trembling went away.

In the year since then, there have been a few adventures. There was the time early on, for example, when I miscalculated how my insulin, my lunch, and getting on a plane would interface, so that my glucose dropped to 50 and there seemed at first to be nothing on the plane to help me raise it. I don't honestly remember what the flight attendant and I came up with, but I did a better job of preparation after that.

At the same time, I've learned by now that there always seems to be someone nearby who recognizes the issue – even from a distance – and appears like magic when I'm starting to lose my grip. A woman in the middle of a meeting who walks over out of nowhere, hands me a package of peanut butter crackers and finds me a few ounces of soda. A guy standing at the counter in the movie complex who sees me run out of a theater with wild eyes and says simply, "Diabetes, right? What do you need?" I tell him and he just buys and hands it to me, saying, "No problem. You okay?" I swear I sometimes feel as if *everybody* is looking out for me.

What they're noticing, of course, at those moments, is the uncontrollable shaking of my hands, but I have signals before that: a little uneasy feeling in my stomach, a warmish flush, my scalp tingling and sweating, and light-headedness, though it doesn't usually get that far with me. I can't risk it. I live alone, go shopping and to the movies alone, travel alone, and typically sleep alone. I have no back-up.

During my first visit to the endocrinologist who put me on insulin, one of his questions was abrupt: "Do you live alone? You know you could die in your sleep."

What he was trying to communicate was that, if my glucose dips low enough while I'm sleeping, if I'm alone, I could slip into a coma and die. I imagine it could happen even with somebody else present. But what usually happens, I'm told, is that the diabetic wakes up agitated, disoriented, and sweating profusely – alone or otherwise. Which I suppose could happen to anyone who's diabetic.

But after I was so unceremoniously presented with the possibility of my own untimely demise and after I spent a couple of weeks taking a hard look at my pillow each night before turning out the light, thinking, "Is tonight perhaps the night...?", I realized that the regimen I was on was unlikely to produce that result – for which I was grateful. I take my long-acting insulin in the morning rather than at bedtime and I check my glucose right before I hit the hay, so if it's under 140, I eat a Greek yogurt and go to bed with the flavor of chocolate or pineapple coconut on my tongue. And on the off-chance I *do* wake up in trouble with my glucose level, I keep a couple of Werther's Originals in the drawer beside my bed. Still – so far – I've woken up every morning glad to see I'm here, a pretty good thought for the first one of the day.

I personally know by now people who have been on insulin for decades and are soldiering on like champs. This helps because I'm still quite new to this party. I'm sure I will learn much more about it over time. But for the purposes of this book, I wanted to get you past the hump of adding insulin to your life in case you freeze up at the thought – like I used to do.

Part 9

What You Plant Grows

Some years ago, when I was far less responsible or spiritually conscious than I try to be today, I had a thought that appeared to be both a carrot and a stick. "The blessing and the curse is this:" it began, "what you plant grows." I wasn't listening to a self-help tape or a sermon. I wasn't in a dungeon or on a retreat. I wasn't going through some agonizing experience that would be sure to mature my soul, if I would let it. I just had the thought and it changed my life.

I immediately began applying it to everything. And I use it in my lectures in classes today because I suspect that it might be the most important truth I ever learned. If I plant beans (I tell my students), I'll get beans. If I come to you with corn and swear I planted beans, you're going to say, "No. You may have *intended* to plant beans. You obviously *thought* you planted beans. You may even want me to *believe* you planted beans. But the fact is: you planted *corn*...because *that's* what grew."

When I first received this tiny, but monumental bit of enlightenment, I applied it to things I should definitely not have been doing. I knew better. It's not just that they were inappropriate or immoral or against the law – it's that they were against my core values and because of that, they were *not* in my best interests. And they brought things into my life that *nobody* would volunteer for. But I was doing them anyway. When I looked at those behaviors from this new perspective, however, I immediately lost the desire to do them. I did not want them growing in the garden of my daily existence. And I was now consciously aware that I was planting them there *myself*.

This might seem like a no-brainer for people that have always done what they know is the right thing to do. But I was not one of those people. Until I had that thought.

I don't know where it came from. And I suspect that there's some version of it in every major religious belief system on the planet. But I couldn't see a way around it. It was a simple fact. And I wasn't going to get into an argument I couldn't win.

My life got a lot simpler and less dramatic after that. At one point, subsequently, when I complained to a friend that I wasn't having fun anymore, his response was telling: "Yeah...and you're not having drama any more either, are you?"

That's been quite some time ago and I still apply this crucial little truth to everything, including managing my diabetes. I can eat whatever I want and it's nobody's business but mine. Yet if I plant foodstuffs and practices that will make me sick rather than healthy, it will soon grow and present itself in my garden in the form of suffering – and I don't want that. If I plant a lot of sitting around instead of physical activity, my garden is soon going to manifest that in the form of diabetic complications that I don't want to experience. If I take a lot of insulin so I can eat unhealthy foods in unhealthy amounts, what I'm doing will shortly be obvious to everyone who sees me – even if they look away and pretend not to notice and even if I loudly claim that I don't *care* what grows in the garden of my life – it's *my* decision!

Nobody wants to suffer. Yet we sometimes plant things emotionally, psychologically, spiritually, and physically that produce exactly that result. And we have a choice.

People in our culture love to quote the verse that reads: "I am the master of my fate, I am the captain of my soul.[i]" But what is the good of that if you run your ship into a rock on purpose? Is it worth it just to prove you have the right? Do you have no more important legacy you want to leave than that you ate and drank whatever you pleased? Do you have no more important purpose than to consume? What do *you* want to grow in the garden of *your* life? And what must you plant to grow it?

---

[i] From "Invictus" by William Ernest Henley.

Appendix

How I Manage My Diabetes Without Health Insurance - - While Going to College Full-Time and Working Two Jobs

by William Schmidt[i]

I'm not writing this is to tell you how terrified I was to find out at 25 that I was diabetic. It's not to talk about the tears that fell when I was struggling to figure out what I could eat or how hearing a doctor say, "You have diabetes," changed my life forever. This book touches on many issues I have personally experienced. Hopefully, you've learned as you read it that life is worth living no matter what and the most important lesson is: "You got this." But I've been asked to tell my story about how a more or less poverty-stricken college student without financial support from friends and family is successfully surviving the struggle of being diabetic while going to college and having to work two jobs.

Before I was diagnosed as diabetic, most people I knew described me as an "over-achiever," but I prefer to say that I just love going to school. I generally took six or seven courses instead of the five most students take and still had a grade point average of nearly straight A's. I took courses all year, including summers, and was on a path to graduate from college with two degrees and two minors in four years. Because of my age, financial aid was providing the assistance I needed so I could simply study and not have to work multiple jobs to pay my bills and college expenses. But all this changed on the day I was told I was diabetic.

The first thing I had to face was that I could no longer continue the fast-paced progression of college I had been following. I had to change habits I had lived by for more than 25 years, including such basics as what I could eat and how to handle my irregular sleeping pattern, two things that finishing college on the fast track had depended on.

At that time, I was spending many late nights (and sometimes early mornings) working to finish writing assignments and study so I could keep making the grades I was making. When I was diagnosed with diabetes, however, I learned that the disease would take a toll on my body if I didn't get enough sleep. I would not only wake up exhausted in the morning, but I would not be able to function the rest of the day. How was I going to make good grades if I couldn't stay up late and couldn't focus during my classes? I had to accept that I would only be able to take a manageable load of school work because, like it or not, my life was different now.

I had always taken as many courses as possible. But, being diagnosed diabetic in the middle of a semester, I had to let go of my pride and drop four of my seven courses. I didn't want to because I knew it would mean being in school for a much longer period of time. But I was not going to let the fact that I couldn't stay up late derail my dream of earning my degree.

I could have given up. I could have said, "College will be too hard because of my new illness; I should just quit." But, our dreams are part of what makes us human. Our dreams give us our own true purpose. And I decided that purpose was worth striving for.

My next challenge was learning what and how to eat. Food is a driving force in my life. Not only does it provide sustenance for survival, but I love to cook. I love making new dishes. I love making the main course for gatherings with other people. But before I was diagnosed diabetic, the schedule I had myself on made it impossible to do any of this. Like many other college students, I would just grab the "quick-fix" of food I needed to keep me going from day to day on the campus.

Sometimes, I thought my only option

was to eat a high-carbohydrate snack on the go. Now, as a diabetic, I had to go out of my way to buy food that was deemed appropriate for my new life, finding "quick-fix" foods I was allowed to eat. And this took some time to figure out. Worse, it was food that made me first realize I now had a financial burden I would have to address in order to keep moving forward.

Buying diabetic-appropriate food to eat is more expensive than buying the food I was used to living on. Thankfully, I had saved as much as I could of my financial aid that semester. So I was able to go to the grocery store and buy what I needed right then. And eventually, I learned how to buy food that was good for me and didn't cost so much. But after that first food shopping spree, I watched my funds disappear at an alarming rate.

I had clung to the hope that I could continue college without being employed. It was a fool's errand, but I held onto that because I knew from previous experience that a job would be time consuming and take away from the hours I need to study. I was determined not to let go of my dream of completing college, but my bank account was making me have doubts.

The final straw came when I went to purchase test strips to check my blood glucose level. I had just spent what seemed like an arm and a leg to get the insulin I needed to stay alive. But the cheapest set of test strips cost sixty dollars for fifty strips or ninety dollars for one hundred. And I broke down in tears right there in the aisle of the store. I knew the better deal was to buy the larger package and I did. But, in the process, I wiped out my savings on barely enough supplies to last a month. I had no idea how I could possibly continue to buy the food, insulin, and test strips I needed, while continuing to go to school.

I had already cut down my courses as far as I could and still maintain my full-time student status so that my financial aid wouldn't come into question. Adding the hassle of not only finding a job, but working at it, seemed an impossible task. I had no idea how I could do it all, but I knew one thing: if I wanted to achieve my dream of getting an education, I had no choice. It would be an uphill battle all the way and I was going to have to fight it.

I had to buy medication and supplies. Insulin was the most expensive item I needed and I knew, with how much I was taking, that I would quickly run out of the first batch I had bought. Diagnosed with a terminal illness as a precondition, I was turned down for every medical insurance policy I applied for. This meant that I had to pay full price for my insulin, which in turn meant that I could barely afford to buy food.

Desperate for relief, I went to the only public health clinic anywhere near where I was living and asked for help. The paperwork and requirements I had to complete even to get a reduced rate on the insulin was almost unbelievable. I would get headaches and leave the building exhausted, faced with returning only a few days later to meet yet another deadline with yet more paperwork. But giving up was not an option. If I had to bend over backwards to get my insulin at a price I could afford, I just had to do it. And it was worth it.

Even so, I needed a cash-flow that my financial aid for school would not provide. To survive, I'd have to get a job and work many hours while still going to class. I didn't have anyone to help me and it was up to me – and only me – to support myself. So, even though I knew it would damage my grades, I went in search of a job.

I used all my resources, talked to all the people I knew, and wound up with two jobs I never thought I would take. One was a job I had quit four years before, swearing I would never go back. And neither was anywhere near glamorous, but I had to swallow my pride once again and take what I could get.

Shortly, I was working as much as sixty hours a week. And just as I feared, my study time vaporized. Working that many hours, I simply didn't have the energy to study. I would fall asleep as soon as I got home, which was probably a good thing anyway because the diabetes made me need my sleep more than ever. I still had the goal of a high grade point average because I had my sights on graduate school and I didn't believe I'd be accepted without making the highest marks possible. But, I learned to be satisfied doing the best I could do. And when I talked to the graduate advisors, I discovered that they were willing to work with me.

Three years later, I am an eligible candidate for graduate school. If I hadn't stayed in school, if I hadn't dropped half of my courses, if I hadn't made peace with the idea that the process was going to take longer than I had hoped, if I hadn't continued to do the best I could despite knowing that my grades were going to fall, and if I hadn't risked humiliation by talking to the graduate advisors about my situation, I would not now be about to graduate with my Bachelor's Degree and continue my education in grad school.

The road is never easy. It seems as if every time I have to renew the paperwork to buy my insulin at a reduced rate, something goes wrong. Maybe they ask for something I think is impossible to get, so the medication is held up, and I have to figure out what to do when I can't get my insulin. I may break down in tears, but I keep pushing forward. I find what I need to produce. I fill out that paperwork. I go above and beyond.

Sometimes, I feel resentful because I don't think we should have to go through all this to get the medication we need to save our lives, but if it is required – as it has been for me – it's worth it. No matter how hopeless the situation seems, I don't give up. I push myself and afterwards, I take that much needed nap or relax doing something enjoyable. I let my dream of my future carry me through the hard times and keep me going.

I've learned to be determined. I've learned to ignore my pride. And I've learned that I am capable of working far harder than I ever wanted to or thought I could. It would be wonderful if life didn't take so much effort, but the truth is, it's often difficult. Still, just like I manage my diabetes, I can manage my life. Some might see that as common sense. Others might never figure it out.

As for me, I've learned to accept the fact that my goals are not going to be handed to me on a silver platter. I knew I wanted to finish college and I was not going to let the financial burdens of becoming diabetic stop me. Looking back on all that I have endured so that I could meet that goal, be accepted into graduate school and finish that, as well, makes me realize that I'm in the process of completing what once seemed like an impossible task. When I was first diagnosed as a diabetic, I honestly thought my dreams were over. I had no money, no one else I could lean on, and no idea where to go from there.

But the end result – who I have become, where I am, and where I'm headed – was worth the fight. It was worth all the tears I've shed. It was worth all the frustration I went through to meet my needs as a diabetic. And it was worth fighting the most difficult battle I will ever fight, the battle that I learned in the end was with myself. It wasn't with my illness. It wasn't with my life circumstances. It was with the fear created by my own thoughts. Life happens; it is what you do after those moments in life that teaches you who you truly are so you can show the world.

My fight is not over. I still have many battles ahead of me, some that I can't even imagine and don't want to. But I will proceed down that dim and uncharted path into my future. I will finish graduate school and afterwards, I will set new goals.

My doctor once told me that I needed to become best friends with my diabetes. And I have. I have found a way to choose my personal path with the ball and chain of a terminal illness attached to my body. Yet even when that weight holds me down, I find a way to keep going forward. My diabetes will not dictate who I will become. I will. And in the end, I will be stronger than I was before, as can you.

---

[i] William Schmidt will graduate in 2016 with a Bachelor of Arts in Psychology and minors in Anthropology and History. He wants to earn a Master's degree next and plans eventually to earn a PhD studying how religion has affected modern U.S. society. He writes articles for the college newspaper and reads comics and novels for fun.

Group Discussion Questions

Part 1 (Mindblown):

1. What did Hensley mean when she said she was lucky to know she was lucky, even though she has diabetes?

2. Are there any ways you have avoided facing the reality of your diagnosis and, if so, how well has that worked out for you?

Part 2 (Weight, Weight – Don't Tell Me!):

1. Hensley writes that her quality of life is about more than being able to drink sweet tea. What is *your* quality of life about?

2. Hensley claims that managing her diabetes is a choice. Do you agree or disagree?

Part 3 (Diabetes Boot Camp):

1. Why does Hensley believe the odds are in a diabetic person's favor when they already have a terminal illness?

2. What were the four main focal points of Hensley's Diabetes Boot Camp routine? Do you focus on all four of them in your life today?

Part 4 (Eating to Live, Not Living to Eat):

1. In the first four paragraphs of this part, Hensley describes the relationship between humans and food. Do you think she's correct and how do you feel about it?

2. What are some of the ways Hensley uses to meet her goal of eating to manage her diabetes? Which ones work for you? Are there any you're not now using that you might try?

Part 5 (To Market, To Market):

1. In this part, Hensley discusses some foods she considers "staples." What are some of your staples and how do you make sure to manage them?

2. What is one of your "guilty pleasures" and how do you negotiate getting to enjoy it without hurting yourself?

Part 6 (Hut! Two, Three, Four!):

1. What are some of the exercise activities Hensley uses to stay fit? What are some of yours?

2. What are some of the ways Hensley builds physical activity into her daily life to help her stay fit? What are some ways you could do the same?

Part 7 (The Tool Kit):

1. Which of the "tools" in Hensley's tool kit do you also have in yours? Which ones

that she mentions might you like to try, if you haven't already?

2. What tools in your tool kit does Hensley *not* discuss?

Part 8 (Takin' My Best Shot):

1. If you're not on insulin already, how do you feel about the possibility that you may someday need to take it?

2. If you *are* on insulin already, what do you like and dislike most about being on it?

Part 9 (What You Plant Grows):

1. What does Hensley mean by writing that "what you plant grows" is both a blessing and a curse?

2. What do you have growing in your garden that you like? Do you have anything growing in your garden you would like to get rid of?

Appendix

1. What were some of the principal changes William had to make in his life to meet his goals after he was diagnosed with diabetes?

2. What are some principal changes you've had to make in your life since you were diagnosed? Are there any others you might need to make?

YOUR LIFE ISN'T OVER

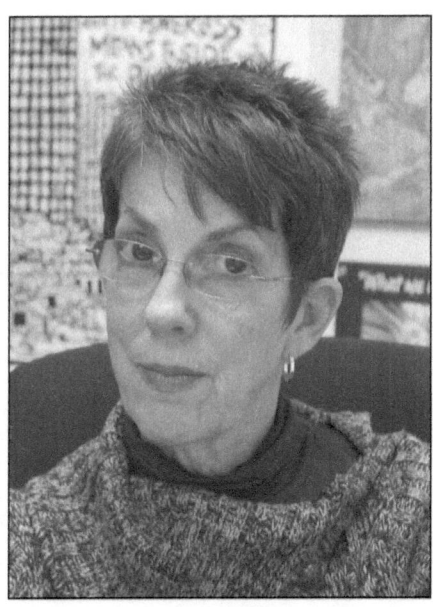

Rebecca Hensley is unapologetic, smart, and wants to change the world. She teaches sociology courses on race, class, gender, and sexuality at a mid-sized public university in the South.

Her blog on race relations (www.WhyAmINotSurprised.blogspot.com) has been visited 425,000 times in nearly 200 countries.

Her blog on in-your-face women (www.inyourfacewomen.blogspot.com) holds 366 mini-bios – one for every day of a year – about women from across time and around the world who did **not** act right.

She expects to soon release an auto-ethnography of her life as a construct to examine race in America. And she works hard to manage her diabetes because she's just warming up.